The GLP-1 Lifestyle: Transform Your Metabolism & Achieve Lasting Weight Loss with or without Semaglutide

Author: Joshua Hackett, M.D.

First Edition: July 2024

Cover Design: Joshua Hackett, M.D.

This book is a work of non-fiction. While the author has made every effort to provide accurate and up-to-date information, the content is for informational purposes only and should not be construed as medical advice. Readers should consult with a healthcare professional for individual medical recommendations.

TABLE OF CONTENTS

Disclaimer I

Introduction II

Section I: The Obesity Crisis **1**

Chapter 1: Theories of Obesity 2

Chapter 2: The Failing State of Weight Loss 9

Chapter 3: GLP-1 To the Rescue? 18

Chapter 4: Semaglutide's Winding History 24

Chapter 5: Stories of Transformation 31

Section II: GLP-1 In Your Body (Physiology) **42**

Chapter 6: The Daily Role of GLP-1 43

Chapter 7: GLP-1 Responds to Nature 51

Chapter 8: GLP-1 Function In Thin People 60

Chapter 9: Powerful Appetite Suppression 64

Chapter 10: Superstar Blood Glucose Levels 72

Chapter 11: The GLP-1 "Slowdown" Effect 78

Section III: Side Effects & Dosing **87**

Chapter 12: My Personal Burning Questions 88

Chapter 13: Common Side Effects 100

Chapter 14: Serious Side Effects 111

Chapter 15: Dosing to Effect 123

Chapter 16: "Mega" Dosing 128

TABLE OF CONTENTS

Chapter 17: "Micro" Dosing 131

Chapter 18: Stopping the Medication, Forever 137

Section IV: Gut Health = Overall Health 143

Chapter 19: Probiotics Matter 144

Chapter 20: Prebiotics Probably Matter More 162

Chapter 21: Postbiotics Might Matter Most 167

Chapter 22: Living In A Rockstar Environment 180

Section V: What's Unique About The GLP-1 Lifestyle? 193

Chapter 23: The Immune-Metabolism Connection 194

Chapter 24: Food & GLP-1 Stimulation 208

Chapter 25: Do You Need to Take Supplements? 220

Section VI: The Lifestyle, Summarized 228

Chapter 26: Now It's Your Turn 229

Conclusion 250

References i

NOTES

DISCLAIMER

The author and publisher disclaim any liability in connection with the use of this information. The recommendations in this book are not intended to replace the advice of a healthcare professional. The reader assumes full responsibility for any decisions made based on the information provided in this book.

The information provided in this book is for educational purposes only. While the strategies and suggestions are based on the latest scientific research and best practices in the field of metabolic health, they are not a substitute for professional medical advice, diagnosis, or treatment.

Always consult with your healthcare provider before starting any new diet, supplement regimen, or exercise program, especially if you have underlying health conditions or are taking medications. By following the recommendations in this book, you accept full responsibility for your health and well-being. Your use of this information is at your own risk, and the author and publisher assume no liability for any potential adverse effects.

INTRODUCTION

Welcome all, if you're holding this book, then very likely you've either embarked on the semaglutide adventure, are considering it, or are interested in boosting your natural "Ozempic-like" weight loss abilities. Good for you for making a choice to change your life and truly make something happen toward your desired weight and metabolic health goals! Many people have jumped into complete darkness with these drugs, experiencing a whirlwind of weight loss, renewed energy, and perhaps a touch of apprehension about what lies beyond the needle (or pill, depending on the drug). I wrote this book to empower readers by showing them that they have control over sustainable long-term weight loss. This means keeping the weight off, improving your metabolic health further over time and enjoying a renewed health-span. Whether you decide to use the help of these medications or not, you will find the answers in these pages.

Imagine having the power to control your appetite, stabilize your blood sugar, and enhance your metabolism. Picture feeling fuller for longer, experiencing fewer cravings, and enjoying sustained energy levels throughout the day. This is the promise of unlocking GLP-1, and this book will show you how. By understanding the science behind GLP-1 and its role in weight regulation, you'll gain a deeper understanding of your own body and its incredible potential for self-healing and transformation. You'll discover that you are not a passive recipient of medication, but an active participant in your own health journey.

fuel your metabolism and work to naturally increase your very own GLP-1 levels. We'll explore and dissect the lifestyle habits that not only aid with the use of GLP-1 receptor agonists, but that allow you to remove them from your life and expect to keep the weight off. For some of you, we will make these medications completely unnecessary to begin with.

I'm here to help you create a life that is vibrant, fulfilling, and free from the shackles of obesity. It's about discovering your own unique path to wellness, embracing a holistic approach to health, where medication is just one tool in the box and at that, hopefully one that gets rusty from lack of use. The ultimate goal is not just weight loss, but a life lived to the fullest.

As you embark on the journey through this book, I want to assure you that your experience will be both enriching and manageable, regardless of your level of scientific expertise or the specific knowledge you seek. This book is designed to be comprehensive yet accessible, allowing you to absorb the information you need without feeling overwhelmed.

First, we will lay the foundation by exploring the obesity crisis and introducing GLP-1 agonist drugs. We delve into the origins and development of these medications, their potential long-term role in managing obesity, and share inspiring (and famous) stories of transformation. This section sets the stage for understanding the broader context and significance of GLP-1 agonists in today's health landscape.

Next, for those interested in a deeper dive into the science, we will provide an in-depth look at the physiology of GLP-1 agonists. We examine the positive effects, side effects, and typical dosing strategies, including microdosing. This section is intended for readers who wish to gain a thorough scientific understanding of how these drugs work within the body. This information was carefully gathered, organized and written to provide a wealth of knowledge found nowhere else. However, I fully understood when writing it that it will go beyond the interest level of many readers. I want to reiterate to you that this is okay! Glean what you personally need to from this book, if the science deep dive doesn't help your journey to health, then skip it.

Then, we will shift our focus to overarching strategies for enhancing health-span through GLP-1. These are broad topics that will completely modernize your knowledge of the body and health. This section could easily be expanded into its own book. I did my best to contain the information and package it neatly into usable facts and reasonable approaches to health. I discuss various approaches to improve overall health and well-being, offering practical advice that can be integrated into your daily life. This section is ideal for readers seeking general strategies to boost their health alongside or independent of GLP-1 agonist use.

Finally, I provide a detailed guide on maximizing the potential of GLP-1, both naturally and through the use of drugs. You will see outlines for specific plans of action, akin to a health coaching plan, to help you achieve optimal results. Whether you are here for comprehensive knowledge or simply seeking actionable steps to enhance your health, this section will provide you with valuable insights and practical tools. I suspect this is the section that many will immediately skip to, again, this is okay!

I understand that each reader comes with unique interests and needs. If you are here specifically for the actionable insights and plans outlined in the final sections, rest assured that you will find them rich with valuable content that makes your time and investment worthwhile. You are welcome to jump directly to that section if it aligns most closely with your goals. However, for a holistic understanding and to fully appreciate the context and depth of the strategies, I encourage you to explore the preceding sections as well.

To support you on your journey, I've created a Facebook group titled "The GLP-1 Lifestyle." This group is tailored specifically to the content of this book, providing a space for you to connect with others, share experiences, ask questions, and receive additional guidance. It's a supportive community where you can find motivation and practical advice from people who are on the same journey as you.

Additionally, I have partnered with Fullscript to offer you convenient access to supplements at a significant discount. We will talk supplements in a later chapter, but suffice to say for now, there are a few that will really help you along your way. First, create a Fullscript account, then sign up with my dispensary and take a look at the template "GLP-1 Lifestyle".

Thank you for joining me on this journey towards better health. Whether you choose to immerse yourself in the detailed science or focus on the practical applications, I hope this book serves as a valuable resource in your pursuit of well-being.

For the Journey,

Dr. Hackett

CHAPTER 1: THEORIES OF OBESITY

ca, the land of opportunity and abundance, has turned these
tes on their heads. We are a society grappling with a not-so-
any-longer epidemic. It's not a virus or a disease, but a
reeping, insidious weight gain that has taken hold of the
(and many other nations around the world). It's a battle
in daily decisions, on gym floors, in the grocery store and at
It's a struggle against biology, environment, and the
ss allure of convenience. The numbers tell a stark story.
)% of American adults are overweight or obese, a statistic
tripled in the last half-century. That's millions of individuals
not just extra pounds, but the health consequences, the
al toll and the societal stigma that often accompany them.

sequences of this obesity epidemic ripple through every
society, exacting a heavy toll on individual lives and the
e system as a whole. Obesity is not merely a cosmetic
it is a major risk factor for a constellation of chronic
that cast a long shadow over our well-being. From type 2
a metabolic disorder characterized by high blood sugar,
ascular diseases like heart attacks and strokes, obesity
ly increases the likelihood of developing these
conditions. Moreover, it elevates the risk of certain
cluding breast, colon, and endometrial cancer, casting
d over the lives of millions. The impact of obesity
yond physical health, eroding quality of life and

SECTION
THE OBES
CRISI

Amer
attribu
silent-
slow-c
nation
fought
home.
relentle
Over 7
that ha
battling
emotion

The con
facet of
healthca
concern;
diseases
diabetes,
to cardio
significan
debilitatin
cancers, i
a dark clo
extends be

shortening lifespan. The excess weight burdens the body, hindering mobility, increasing the risk of injuries, and contributing to chronic pain. It can lead to sleep apnea, a disorder characterized by disrupted breathing during sleep, further compromising overall health and well-being. The emotional toll of obesity is equally significant, with individuals often facing stigma, discrimination, and a diminished sense of self-worth.

Why are weight issues such an uphill battle for so many? Why has it become so prevalent and insidious? It's not simply a lack of willpower or a failure of character. The science of weight regulation is complex, a delicate dance of hormones, genetics, and environmental influences. Our bodies are wired to conserve energy, a survival mechanism from our hunter-gatherer ancestors that now works against us in a world of abundance. Our bodies are meant to move, be one with our environments, and have many hours of relaxation, plus 8 hours of sleep every night. Many of you are now thinking, "as if"! This is of course the problem and a 30,000 foot view of it at that. Let's drop altitude a bit and take a look at some theories of obesity.

First, we have the traditional calorie imbalance theory, which, while partially true, doesn't capture the full picture. The calorie imbalance theory posits that weight gain occurs when we consume more calories than we expend. This straightforward equation of energy balance—calories from food and beverages as 'input' and calories burned through metabolism and physical activity as 'output'—suggests that surplus energy is stored as fat, leading to weight gain. Conversely, a calorie deficit results in the breakdown of stored fat for energy, leading to weight loss. However, this 'calories in, calories out' (CICO) model doesn't tell the whole story. Our bodies are not simple calculators, and calories are not created equal. The quality of our food choices, the composition of our diet, and our individual metabolic rates all play a role in how our bodies process and utilize energy.

Next, let's explore the hormonal imbalance theory. This theory posits that when certain hormones are out of balance, they can trigger a cascade of events that promote weight gain. Leptin, known as the "satiety hormone," is produced by fat cells and signals to the brain that we're full and should stop eating. However, some individuals develop leptin resistance, in which the brain no longer responds effectively to leptin's signals, leading to persistent hunger and overeating despite adequate caloric intake. Ghrelin, the "hunger hormone" produced in the stomach, plays a crucial role by stimulating appetite. When ghrelin levels remain elevated, even after eating, it can result in increased cravings and overeating. As you may have guessed, these hormones are often deranged in the modern, overweight human.

Another key hormone implicated in this theory is insulin, which regulates blood sugar levels. Insulin resistance (IR), a condition where the body's cells become less responsive to insulin, is commonly associated with obesity. This resistance can lead to elevated blood sugar levels, increased fat storage, and further hormonal disruptions. In addition to leptin, ghrelin, and insulin, hormones like cortisol, which is released in response to stress, can also impact weight by promoting fat storage and increasing appetite.

Insulin resistance (IR) is a critical factor in the development of obesity and metabolic disorders. When cells in the body become less responsive to insulin, it leads to higher blood sugar levels and increased fat storage. This condition is often a precursor to type 2 diabetes and is intricately linked with metabolic disease.

Polycystic Ovary Syndrome (PCOS) is another condition that is strongly associated with insulin resistance. IR and PCOS go hand in hand and is a characteristic feature of PCOS. This exacerbates symptoms of the syndrome, including weight gain, irregular menstrual cycles, and fertility issues. Throughout this book, when we discuss insulin resistance, it's important to recognize that many of the principles and treatments apply directly to managing PCOS as well. Anytime you see IR mentioned, you can assume that these insights are also relevant to PCOS management.

While the calorie imbalance theory focuses on the quantity of calories consumed and expended, the hormonal imbalance theory emphasizes the quality of those calories and their impact on hormonal signaling. Diets high in processed foods, refined sugars, and unhealthy fats can cause spikes in insulin and disrupt the balance of leptin, ghrelin, and other hormones. This disruption can create a vicious cycle of cravings, overeating, and weight gain. Understanding the hormonal basis of weight gain offers new avenues for treatment and prevention and sophisticates our approach.

Moving on, we have the emerging gut microbiome theory. This offers a fascinating and novel perspective on the obesity epidemic, shifting the focus from calories and hormones to the trillions of microorganisms residing in our digestive tracts. This theory proposes that the composition and diversity of our gut microbiome, the vast community of bacteria, viruses, fungi, and other microbes that call our intestines home, may play a significant role in weight regulation and metabolic health. Research suggests that individuals with obesity often have a less diverse gut microbiome compared to those with healthy weights.

Certain types of bacteria, such as Firmicutes, are more abundant in individuals with obesity, while others, like Bifidobacterium spp., are less prevalent. This imbalance in gut bacteria may contribute to increased energy extraction from food, altered fat metabolism, and inflammation, all of which can contribute to weight gain and metabolic dysfunction.

The gut microbiome is not a passive bystander in the weight gain process. It actively communicates with our bodies, influencing hormone production, immune function, and even brain activity. Studies have shown that gut bacteria can produce metabolites impacting appetite regulation, insulin sensitivity, and fat storage. They can also influence hormones like leptin and ghrelin, contributing to the complex interplay of factors determining our weight. This means the microbiome theory encompasses the previous theories we've discussed. The implications of this theory are far-reaching. While research is ongoing, it offers a tantalizing glimpse into the intricate connection between our gut health and our weight. We will dive deeply into the health of our guts in later chapters.

Next, we must discuss the lifestyle theory of obesity. Most specifically, I want to discuss the important topics of stress and sleep. Chronic stress often leads to poor sleep quality and duration, which in turn disrupts the regulation of hunger hormones like ghrelin and leptin, increasing appetite and cravings for high-calorie foods. Moreover, insufficient sleep impairs cognitive function and decision-making, making it harder to resist unhealthy food choices and maintain a balanced diet. This combination of chronic stress and inadequate sleep perpetuates a vicious cycle that exacerbates weight gain and undermines efforts to achieve and maintain a healthy weight.

und consequences for our weight and overall health. arch shows that insufficient sleep disrupts hormone balance, ases appetite, and impairs glucose metabolism. The true t of this sleep deprivation epidemic is hard to quantify, as our tive sleep habits have shifted so dramatically that we've lost with what truly restful sleep feels like. What we consider al" sleep may be far from optimal, leaving us perpetually ed, irritable, and vulnerable to weight gain. Our environment, s a powerful force in the weight loss struggle, a constant e of temptations and obstacles. It's a world where biological oositions are amplified, and healthy choices become singly difficult. But while we cannot change our genes or tely escape our environment, we can arm ourselves with dge, develop coping strategies, and make conscious to navigate this challenging landscape.

esity epidemic is a multifaceted problem with far-reaching uences. It's a public health crisis that demands urgent n and innovative solutions. As we grapple with the al, environmental, and behavioral factors contributing to we must also address its economic and social costs. The of obesity is not just a personal struggle; it's a societal e requiring a comprehensive and collaborative approach ntion, treatment, and support. Traditional weight loss nes often fall short in the face of such a complex problem. o reimagine our strategies, embracing a holistic nding of the factors that contribute to weight gain and innovative solutions that address the root causes of

Our modern environment has placed unprec
our bodies, unlike anything experienced in th
years of human history. This rapid accelerat
factors over the last century has taken a sig
health. While the effects of stress are well-c
on obesity remains a topic of debate and c
mistake, however; this modern-day scourg
balance, notably increasing cortisol levels
resulting in numerous adverse effects. Thi
lead to heightened appetite, cravings for
diminished ability to feel full. Essentially,
formidable ally in weight gain, thwarting
healthy weight.

Stress has become a constant compani
of us cope in unhealthy ways, such as t
and alcohol for temporary relief. This be
matter of poor choices but a deeply ing
response. Carbohydrates, especially th
processed foods, trigger the release o
neurotransmitter associated with moo
Similarly, alcohol can initially reduce a
relaxation. However, these short-term
term cost. Ironically, our attempts to
perpetuate the cycle of weight gain a

Poor sleep is another major health c
contributor to obesity. Our days are
artificial light, endless to-do lists, ar
of which interfere with our natural s
many of us are chronically sleep-d

prof
Rese
incre
exte
colle
touch
"norm
fatigu
then,
barrag
predis
increa
compl
knowle
choice

The ob
conseq
attentio
biologic
obesity,
burden
challeng
to preve
approac
It's time
understa
exploring
obesity.

CHAPTER 2: THE FAILING STATE OF WEIGHT LOSS

The weight loss rollercoaster continues its relentless cycle. We embark on restrictive diets, endure grueling workouts, and white-knuckle our way through cravings, only to find ourselves back at square one, the weight creeping back on, our spirits deflated. It's a frustrating and demoralizing experience, one that leaves many feeling defeated and questioning their willpower. But, what if the problem isn't simply a lack of willpower or discipline? We know from Chapter 1 that the weight loss struggle is a symptom of a deeper issue, a complex interplay of biological, psychological, and environmental factors that have been overlooked or misunderstood.

This chapter will delve into the heart of this complex issue, exploring the reasons why weight loss is so difficult for so many. We will examine the calorie conundrum, the macronutrient maze, the allure of fad diets, the role of exercise, and the emotional underpinnings of eating behaviors. We'll challenge conventional wisdom, debunk myths, and offer a fresh perspective on the weight loss journey. By understanding the root causes of our struggles, we can break free from the cycle of failure and embark on a path toward sustainable weight loss and lasting health. We'll discover that weight loss is not just about counting calories or restricting food groups; it's about nourishing our bodies, understanding our unique needs, and cultivating a healthy relationship with food, amongst (many) other strategies!

The weight loss landscape is littered with the wreckage of failed diets, a testament to the enduring struggle against excess weight. The prevailing narrative often casts this struggle as a simple equation from which we are already familiar: calories in versus calories out. Eat less, move more, and the pounds will melt away. The calorie conundrum is a battleground where willpower clashes with biology. We are bombarded with messages about calorie counting, portion control, and the importance of maintaining a calorie deficit. Yet, despite our best intentions, our bodies often rebel, clinging to fat stores and resisting our efforts to shed them. This is a design of the wisest variety, straight from nature.

This rebellion is not a sign of weakness or a lack of discipline; it's a reflection of our evolutionary heritage. Though we know it is only a part of the puzzle, it is important that you understand how best to utilize calories and their constituents, the macronutrients.

Macronutrients are the cornerstone of human metabolism, serving as primary sources of energy and essential building blocks for the body. They are divided into three main categories: carbohydrates, proteins, and fats. Each macronutrient plays a vital role in maintaining health and supporting metabolic processes. Carbohydrates fuel cellular activities, especially in the brain and muscles. Proteins, composed of amino acids, are essential for muscle repair, immune function, and the synthesis of enzymes and hormones. Fats, a dense energy source, are necessary for the absorption of fat-soluble vitamins, hormone production, and cell membrane integrity. Let's dig in a bit.

Carbohydrates, often demonized in the weight loss world, are the body's primary source of energy. They are broken down into glucose, which fuels our cells and powers our activities. However, not all carbohydrates are created equal. Refined carbohydrates, found in processed foods and sugary drinks, can cause rapid spikes in blood sugar levels, followed by crashes that leave us feeling tired and hungry. These fluctuations can disrupt our hormonal balance, trigger cravings, and contribute to weight gain. These are known as simple sugars and have a high "glycemic index," which is essentially a food's ability to raise your blood sugar. On the other hand, complex carbohydrates, found in whole grains, fruits, and vegetables, are digested more slowly, providing sustained energy and promoting stable blood sugar levels. This defines a lower glycemic index. Also, as very importantly, complex carbs are our most significant source of fiber. Fiber has been shown time and time again to be one of the healthiest food items that we can consume, period. The "why" here is quite simple; fiber feeds the gut. Given the emergence of knowledge surrounding the gut microbiome and its critical importance to our health, you can now understand that connection. Fiber also appears to have direct effects on GLP-1 production. Amazing stuff!

Protein, the building block of muscle and tissue, is another essential macronutrient for weight loss. It promotes satiety, the feeling of fullness, and helps preserve muscle mass during weight loss, which is crucial for maintaining a healthy metabolism. Inadequate protein intake can lead to muscle loss, a slower metabolism, and difficulty maintaining weight loss in the long run. High-protein diets enhance satiety and support weight loss, working synergistically with the benefits of GLP-1 agonists in regulating appetite and promoting metabolic health.

Fat, seriously vilified in the past and moderately vilified today, is now recognized as an essential nutrient for optimal health. It provides energy, supports hormone production, and helps us absorb fat-soluble vitamins. There is still controversy surrounding what a "good" or "bad" fat actually constitutes. What I will tell you for the purposes of this book and for your health span is that trans fats, overabundance of omega 6 fatty acids and oxidized (over-heated) fats are doing you zero favors. Ditch them. Healthy fats can promote satiety, reduce inflammation, and support cardiovascular health. Omega-3 fatty acids, a type of polyunsaturated fat, are particularly beneficial for reducing inflammation and supporting cardiovascular health, complementing the metabolic benefits of GLP-1 agonists.

Balancing macronutrient intake is crucial for maintaining metabolic health, managing weight, and preventing chronic diseases. Each macronutrient influences metabolic processes differently and interacts with hormonal regulators, including GLP-1. However, macronutrient ratios get confusing, really fast. In fact, they are the basis for a large number of trendy or so called "fad" diets (think low carb high fat, or LCHF). We will discuss specific ratios and strategies later; it really doesn't need to be as complicated as presented by many trends today. What is more important is our modern food environment, a landscape saturated with highly processed, calorie-dense foods designed to hijack our taste buds and trigger cravings. These foods, often low in nutrients and high in sugar, ugly fats and salt, can disrupt our hormonal balance, promote inflammation, and sabotage our weight loss efforts.

The key to navigating the macronutrient maze is to find a balance. There is no one-size-fits-all approach, and the ideal macronutrient ratio can vary depending on your activity level, metabolic health, and personal goals. However, some general guidelines can be helpful. A balanced diet typically includes a moderate amount of complex carbohydrates, more protein than most people recommend and a moderate amount of healthy fats. But we'll more into these ratios later.

Fad diets often present themselves as a beacon, promising a swift and effortless journey to a slimmer, healthier you. Their alluring claims attract people in droves. Guarantees of rapid weight loss, detoxification and miraculous transformations tap into our deepest desires for a quick fix, a shortcut to the body of our dreams. But like the siren songs of Greek mythology, fad diets often lead their followers astray, luring them into a treacherous sea of deprivation, nutritional deficiencies, and, ultimately, rebound weight gain. These diets, with their rigid rules and restrictive food lists, may offer temporary results, but they are rarely sustainable in the long run.

Many of these diets are based on flawed science or anecdotal evidence ("guru" science, quite often). They often demonize entire food groups and therefore the opposing trend diet. This leads to imbalanced nutrition, deficiencies and stress on the body, as if you needed more. Their restrictive nature can trigger cravings, binge eating, and a rebound effect where we regain the lost weight, often with a few extra pounds added on for good measure. The low-carb craze, for example, has swept the nation in recent years, promising rapid weight loss and improved metabolic health. While there is evidence to support reducing refined carbohydrates and added sugars, many low-carb diets go to extremes by eliminating entire food groups like fruits and whole grains, leading to the issues described previously. Folks, plain and simple, they are called fad diets for a reason, and likely many of the ones you've tried in the past fall firmly into this category!

Exercise is often the focus of weight loss strategies and is frequently taken to extreme levels. I struggle to write these next paragraphs because I truly believe in the power of exercise. It's important, however, that you understand that, like all else, exercise needs to be balanced with your current abilities, your goals and the current status of your health.

Exercise approached without balance or consideration for individual circumstances can become counterproductive, even harmful. Put simply, stressed out, inflamed and out of shape individuals should not start doing Cross-fit tomorrow morning. There is a vicious cycle at play when a chronically stressed and chronically inflamed individual engages in grueling, high-intensity exercise. The intention to lose weight and improve health can ironically lead to exacerbated stress levels and metabolic issues. For many modern humans, the addition of intense exercise amplifies the production of cortisol, the body's primary stress hormone. Elevated cortisol levels, when sustained over time, is completely destructive to health, laying waste to immune function, fat burning (particularly in the abdominal area), and sleep. This hormonal imbalance creates a paradox where the very act of exercising, meant to reduce weight and improve health, ends up undermining these goals. Sleep problems and metabolic derangement follow, and the vicious cycle spins out of control.

In light of these considerations, it is crucial to adopt a balanced approach to exercise. This means tailoring workouts to individual fitness levels, health conditions, and stress levels. First incorporating low intensity activities like walking can provide the benefits of exercise without overwhelming the body's stress response systems. Listening to the body and prioritizing rest and recovery is equally important. Ultimately, the goal should be to integrate exercise as a sustainable, enjoyable part of a holistic health strategy, rather than a punishing regimen that may do more harm than good.

I do want to mention that a long term goal is to get yourself to a point where intense exercise is a smart goal that elevates your wellness. Exercise is a powerful catalyst for metabolic transformation. Think of exercise as a celebration of your body's incredible capabilities. It's a way to tap into your inner strength, push your limits, and discover the joy of movement. Exercise has profound effects that I'll only touch on here, such as very significant, positive impacts on insulin sensitivity, a key factor in metabolic health, as well as offering a strong metabolism boost, the rate at which your body burns calories. Exercise also increases your muscle mass. Muscle is a metabolic organ all on its own and offers profound benefits to metabolic optimization. Not to mention exercise is a serious mood booster, confidence builder and social outlet. Take that vicious cycle and reverse it. It simply improves lives.

The battle for weight loss is not solely waged on the physical battlefield of calories and exercise; it's a deeply personal struggle that unfolds in the theater of the mind. Emotions, those powerful currents that surge through our lives, can often hijack our eating behaviors, leading us down a treacherous path of overindulgence and self-sabotage. Emotional eating, a coping mechanism as old as time, is a complex and often misunderstood phenomenon. It's not simply a matter of willpower or lack of discipline; it's a deeply ingrained response to stress, anxiety, boredom, loneliness, and a myriad of other emotions that we may struggle to process or express.

In the throes of emotional turmoil, food can offer a temporary solace, a fleeting escape from the pain and discomfort of our inner world. The sweet embrace of chocolate, the salty crunch of chips, the comforting warmth of a bowl of pasta—these culinary delights can momentarily numb our emotions, providing a brief respite from the storm raging within. This emotional refuge comes at a cost. The calories from these comfort foods add up quickly, the resulting blood sugar spikes and crashes can further exacerbate mood swings and cravings and oftentimes, these binges coincide with times of sedentary behavior, high stress and poor sleep. Here we are back to that vicious cycle. Are you starting to see how these life cycles can play out over years or decades?

There is one last, depressing fact that I want to address now: 95% of weight lost is regained. Are you kidding me?! All these setbacks, all these issues and considerations, only to have success stolen from the vast majority of people successful in losing weight. The reality of this is relatively unknown, but I want to quickly share it with you now (we will devote a chapter to this later): fat loss hurts your body. Fat loss causes an injury response and your body and immune system respond, thinking they are doing you a favor by getting back those precious resources. An important part of this book is introducing you to the concepts of "immune centric fat loss", dubbed by my friend Joel Greene. We must offset the injury of fat loss and leave the body feeling secure with its new lack of fat store resources!

The weight loss journey is a complex and often challenging endeavor, fraught with obstacles and setbacks. It's married to confusion, best friends with deception and laced with charlatans. It's an arduous journey, one where most people struggle for years just to find a trailhead (and usually a wrong one, at that). The weight loss journey is not a one-size-fits-all endeavor, clearly. It's a deeply personal and individualized process that requires a holistic approach, one that addresses all aspects of weight loss and sustainability in keeping the weight off. It is a daunting challenge, but one you are fully capable of conquering!

CHAPTER 3: GLP-1 TO THE RESCUE?

Amidst this landscape of struggle and complexity, a new beacon of hope has emerged on the weight loss horizon. The "semaglutides", or GLP-1 receptor agonists, have hit mainstream in a big way. Throughout this book, I will be referring to GLP-1 receptor agonists like Ozempic, Wegovy and Rybelsus, as well as non-semaglutide drugs like Mounjaro (tirzepatide), as simply "semaglutide", to simplify the matter. Semaglutide is a medication initially designed to treat type 2 diabetes, but has shown remarkable promise in helping individuals shed excess pounds and reclaim their health. Semaglutide doesn't rely on traditional diets and exercise programs, those fraught with so many issues we discussed in the previous chapter. Semaglutide works by harnessing the power of our own biology, targeting the hormonal imbalances and physiological mechanisms that contribute to weight gain. At least that's what the commercials want you to believe. Of course, part is true, part is false, and part is unknown.

At the heart of semaglutide's transformative potential lies GLP-1, short for glucagon-like peptide-1 (I'll keep it short throughout the book!), a naturally occurring hormone. Semaglutide actually functions to occupy GLP-1 receptors, meaning that it mimics the hormone within the body, signaling to our body that GLP-1 is elevated. GLP-1 plays a crucial role in our bodies' intricate energy balance system and is a gut hormone released in response to food intake. It acts as a messenger, communicating with various organs and systems to regulate appetite, blood sugar levels, and digestion.

When GLP-1 docks at its receptor, it sets off a cascade of events that tell your brain, "You're full, satisfied and can put down the fork." This gentle nudge towards satiety helps you eat less, curb cravings, and maintain a healthy weight. Different levels of fullness, or satiety, have different strengths of signaling for GLP-1 release, which acts directly in the brain to target specific areas that control appetite and food intake. When GLP-1 levels rise, these receptors are activated, sending a message to the brain that we've had enough to eat. This leads to a decrease in hunger and cravings, making it easier to resist the urge to overindulge.

In recent years, blood glucose regulation has become a focal point for many health-conscious individuals. It's not uncommon to see people, even those without diabetes, using continuous glucose monitors and apps to track their glucose responses to different foods. This trend underscores the growing awareness of the importance of optimizing food intake, digestion, and glucose metabolism. GLP-1 significantly contributes to this process by stimulating insulin release from the pancreas. Insulin is the primary hormone responsible for transporting glucose from the bloodstream into cells. A deficiency in insulin production or a decrease in its effectiveness is what characterizes type 1 and type 2 diabetes, respectively. Concurrently, GLP-1 suppresses glucagon release, a hormone that raises blood sugar levels. This dual regulatory action by GLP-1 helps maintain steady blood sugar levels, thereby preventing the spikes and crashes that can lead to fatigue, cravings, and long-term health issues like type 2 diabetes.

GLP-1 doesn't stop there. Digestive rate and capability has a powerful effect on nutrient uptake, blood glucose regulation and overall health. GLP-1 influences digestion by slowing down the rate at which food leaves the stomach. This "delayed gastric emptying" prolongs the feeling of fullness, further contributing to reduced calorie intake. There is evidence to suggest that this decreased motility even allows for more nutrient absorption in the small intestine!

By promoting satiety, regulating blood sugar, and slowing digestion, you may begin to understand just how powerful GLP-1 acts as an ally in the quest for weight loss and metabolic health. Semaglutide is more than just a weight loss drug. It's a potential game-changer for individuals struggling with metabolic syndrome, obesity and their associated health risks. Rigorous clinical trials have consistently demonstrated semaglutide's abilities. In the *SUSTAIN 6* study, for example, participants taking Ozempic experienced an average reduction in HbA1c[1] of 1.2-1.8%, a clinically significant improvement.

Semaglutide has also been shown to reduce the risk of major cardiovascular events, such as heart attacks, strokes, and cardiovascular death, in people with type 2 diabetes and established cardiovascular disease. This cardio-protective effect is likely due to semaglutide's ability to lower blood pressure and improve levels of chronic inflammation, two key risk factors for heart disease. In the *REWIND* trial, semaglutide was associated with a 26% reduction in major adverse cardiovascular events, a remarkable finding that underscores its potential to improve both

---

1 HbA1c is a measure of long term blood glucose and currently the best result we have to track chronic sustained blood sugar levels.

metabolic and cardiovascular health. These benefits extend to other organs as well. Semaglutide has been shown to protect against diabetic kidney disease, a common complication of diabetes that can lead to kidney failure. In the *SUSTAIN 6* study, semaglutide reduced the risk of kidney disease progression by 36%, a significant finding for individuals with diabetes who are at increased risk of kidney damage.

These compelling clinical trial results highlight semaglutide's potential to transform the lives of individuals with type 2 diabetes and metabolic syndrome. By improving blood sugar control, reducing cardiovascular risk, and protecting against kidney disease, Ozempic offers a comprehensive approach to managing this complex condition and improving long-term health outcomes.

While semaglutide's potential is undeniable, it's crucial to approach it with discernment and a holistic perspective. As a practitioner deeply rooted in the principles of natural health and wellness, I firmly believe that optimizing your body's innate GLP-1 production should be the first line of defense in the battle against weight gain and metabolic dysfunction. Semaglutide sheds light on the potential of GLP-1 in optimizing our health. We can optimize our natural GLP-1 production through a combination of lifestyle modifications which we will discuss later. By holding this book, you are well on your way to utilizing your natural GLP-1 response.

We must recognize that there are individuals for whom these lifestyle modifications alone may not be enough. For those who have struggled with obesity for years, who have tried countless diets and exercise programs to no avail, semaglutide can offer a much-needed lifeline. It can jumpstart weight loss, break through plateaus, and provide a renewed sense of hope and motivation.

However, semaglutide is not magic, and it should not be viewed as a long-term solution. It's a powerful tool, but like any tool, it must be used with care and intention. It's a temporary bridge, not a permanent dwelling. The goal is to utilize semaglutide as a catalyst for change, a springboard to a healthier lifestyle that can be sustained even after the medication is discontinued. This means that semaglutide is most appropriate for individuals who are committed to making lasting changes to their diet, exercise habits, and overall lifestyle. It's for those who are willing to put in the work, to embrace a holistic approach to health, and to view the drug as a stepping stone on their journey, not the final destination.

Semaglutide is heralding a new era in the weight loss landscape, shifting the conversation away from restrictive diets and grueling exercise regimes towards a more nuanced understanding of the biological underpinnings of weight gain. Part of this shift was a requirement that needed to happen. Gone should be the days of punishing workouts and starving levels of calorie deficits. These do not work and in fact do a lot of damage! We will dive into why this is the case in a later chapter. We are seeing a paradigm shift that acknowledges the complex interplay that occurs with healthy weight loss. This is an offering of a potential solution that goes beyond suffering, yo-yo dieting and chronic weight struggles. Semaglutide's success in clinical trials and real-world settings has sparked a renewed sense of hope for individuals struggling with weight loss. It has demonstrated that weight management is not solely a matter of individual effort, but also a biological challenge that can be addressed with targeted interventions. This new understanding has opened up a world of possibilities for those who have previously felt trapped in a cycle of failed diets and frustrated attempts at weight loss.

The debate surrounding semaglutide's role in the weight loss journey is far from settled. It's a complex issue with no easy answers, a reflection of the multifaceted nature of obesity itself. But one thing is certain: semaglutide has ignited a conversation, a dialogue that challenges our assumptions about weight loss and forces us to confront the limitations of traditional approaches. It's a conversation that will continue to evolve as we delve deeper into the science, the ethics, and the lived experiences of those who have embarked on this new path to wellness. Semaglutide has opened our eyes to the role that hormones can play in weight loss and offers a sneak peak into the future of obesity medicine, one where we are more aware and savvy of the options to optimize these hormones. The promise of semaglutide is not merely about shedding pounds; it's about breaking down barriers, challenging stigmas, and empowering individuals to take control of their health. It's about opening up new possibilities, new conversations, and a new era in the ongoing quest for a healthier, happier life.

CHAPTER 4: SEMAGLUTIDE'S WINDING HISTORY

Semaglutide's success story is rooted in a fascinating journey of scientific and medical innovation. Scientists had long recognized the potential of targeting GLP-1 for diabetes management, yet early efforts were stymied by the hormone's rapid degradation in the body. The short half-life of native GLP-1 meant it was quickly broken down before delivering substantial therapeutic benefits, a significant hurdle for early adopters and developers of these novel therapeutic agents.

The exploration of GLP-1's potential began in the 1980s, when researchers first identified its role in glucose metabolism. GLP-1 was found to enhance insulin secretion in response to food intake, inhibit glucagon release, and slow gastric emptying, all of which contributed to better glycemic control. Despite these promising properties, the clinical application of GLP-1 was initially limited due to its short half-life, lasting only a few minutes in the bloodstream before being degraded by the enzyme dipeptidyl peptidase-4 (DPP-4).

In the 1990s, researchers were determined to overcome the rapid degradation of native GLP-1 in the body, which led to the development of GLP-1 receptor agonists. These compounds were designed to mimic the beneficial actions of GLP-1 but with longer-lasting effects, making them more practical for therapeutic use. A significant breakthrough came with the discovery of exendin-4, a peptide found in the saliva of the Gila monster, which captivated scientists, given its unique properties and remarkable similarity to GLP-1. This discovery, seemingly plucked from the realm of the improbable, provided a pivotal breakthrough in diabetes treatment. Unlike native GLP-1, exendin-4 exhibited a remarkable resistance to this enzymatic breakdown. This resistance grants it a much longer half-life in the bloodstream, making it far more suitable for therapeutic use. The peptide's stability and prolonged action meant that it could provide these benefits with less frequent dosing, a significant advantage over native GLP-1. This led to the development of exenatide, a synthetic version of exendin-4, which was approved by the FDA in 2005 and marketed as Byetta. Exenatide's introduction marked a significant leap forward in diabetes management, offering patients a more practical and effective means of controlling their blood sugar levels. The journey from the venomous saliva of a desert-dwelling lizard to a groundbreaking diabetes treatment underscores the unpredictable path of scientific discovery.

Patients using exenatide experienced significant improvements in HbA1c levels and many reported weight loss. Exenatide ushered in a new era of innovation in diabetes management, characterized by a better understanding of the incretin system and its therapeutic potential. Following this breakthrough, liraglutide (marketed as Victoza) emerged as another significant milestone in the realm of GLP-1 receptor agonist therapy. Approved by the FDA in 2010, liraglutide was designed with a unique structural modification: a fatty acid side chain that enabled it to bind to albumin, a protein in the blood. The fatty acid side chain not only prolongs the hormone's activity but also ensures a steady and sustained effect throughout the day.

This new innovation extended liraglutide's half-life, allowing for once-daily dosing, a considerable improvement in convenience over previous treatments. The clinical trials leading up to liraglutide's approval demonstrated its impressive efficacy in managing blood sugar levels and promoting weight loss. Patients with type 2 diabetes who were treated with liraglutide also experienced significant reductions in HbA1c and weight loss.

The success of liraglutide again significantly impacted the diabetes treatment landscape, making it a popular choice among both patients and healthcare providers. Its once-daily dosing regimen improved adherence and provided patients with a more manageable treatment option. Beyond its glucose-lowering effects, liraglutide's capacity to aid in weight reduction added a valuable therapeutic benefit, further solidifying its role in comprehensive diabetes care. Despite these successes, the search for even more effective and convenient therapies continued. Researchers aimed to develop GLP-1 receptor agonists that could be administered less frequently while providing superior efficacy and tolerability. This quest led to the development of semaglutide, a once-weekly version with an even longer half-life than its predecessors. Semaglutide's innovative formulation involved amino acid substitutions and the addition of a spacer and fatty acid side chain, enhancing its stability and binding affinity with albumin. Semaglutide was first approved by the FDA in 2017 under the brand name Ozempic for the treatment of type 2 diabetes. Its approval was based on a series of robust clinical trials that highlighted its remarkable ability to improve glycemic control and induce significant weight loss.

The success of semaglutide in diabetes management quickly spurred interest in its potential for weight loss in individuals without diabetes. Researchers and healthcare professionals were intrigued by the significant weight loss observed as a secondary benefit in patients. Clinical trials designed to specifically investigate semaglutide's efficacy for weight management began to yield promising results, capturing the attention of the broader medical community and regulatory agencies. One of the pivotal studies in this context was the *STEP (Semaglutide Treatment Effect in People with Obesity)* program, which encompassed a series of trials aimed at evaluating the impact of semaglutide on weight loss in non-diabetic individuals. The results were impressive. Participants who received semaglutide experienced substantial reductions in body weight, with many achieving clinically significant weight loss of 15% or more. These outcomes were accompanied by improvements in various metabolic markers, such as blood pressure, lipid profiles, and inflammatory markers, underscoring the comprehensive health benefits of GLP-1.

Another notable development in the GLP-1 receptor agonist family was the introduction of Rybelsus, an oral formulation of semaglutide approved by the FDA in 2019. Unlike its injectable counterparts, Rybelsus offered the convenience of a once-daily oral tablet, making it an attractive option for patients who preferred to avoid injections. The development of Rybelsus involved sophisticated pharmaceutical technologies to ensure the stability and absorption of semaglutide in the gastrointestinal tract. Rybelsus is yet another innovative addition to the GLP-1 receptor agonist family and the only oral formulation currently available.

Despite the convenience of Rybelsus, Ozempic remains highly popular due to its strong efficacy in both blood sugar control and cardiovascular risk reduction. Both medications have shown effectiveness in lowering HbA1c levels and promoting weight loss. In clinical comparisons, patients taking 1 mg of Ozempic typically achieve a slightly higher reduction in HbA1c (around 1.6%) compared to those taking 14 mg of Rybelsus (a comparable dose). This marginal difference, along with the cardiovascular benefits, keeps Ozempic a preferred option for many patients and healthcare providers. Research didn't stop there, however.

In 2021, semaglutide was approved for chronic weight management under the brand name Wegovy. Administering Wegovy involves a straightforward process, identical to Ozempic. Patients inject the medication subcutaneously in the abdomen, thigh, or upper arm, once per week. This expansion into weight management marked a significant milestone, demonstrating the versatility and broad therapeutic potential of GLP-1 receptor agonists. It was first approved by the FDA on June 4, 2021, for adults with obesity or overweight individuals with at least one weight-related condition, such as high blood pressure, type 2 diabetes, or high cholesterol. The approval of Wegovy was built on the strong foundation of semaglutide's success in managing type 2 diabetes. Clinical trials, particularly the *STEP (Semaglutide Treatment Effect in People with Obesity)* program, played a pivotal role in demonstrating its efficacy. These trials revealed that participants taking Wegovy experienced significant weight loss, averaging around 12.4% of their initial body weight compared to those on placebo, who lost only about 2.4%.

The FDA's approval of Wegovy for weight management was followed by another significant milestone in 2024, when it was approved for reducing the risk of major adverse cardiovascular events (MACE) in people with cardiovascular disease and either obesity or overweight. This approval was based on the *SELECT* trial, which included over 17,000 participants and showed that semaglutide reduced the risk of cardiovascular death, non-fatal myocardial infarction, and non-fatal stroke by 20% compared to placebo.

Approved by the FDA in 2022, the newest member on the market, Mounjaro (tirzepatide), is unique as it is the first dual glucose-dependent insulinotropic polypeptide (GIP) and GLP-1 receptor agonist medication. This dual action mechanism allows Mounjaro to offer unparalleled efficacy in glycemic control and weight reduction compared to traditional GLP-1 receptor agonists like semaglutide.

Tirzepatide leads to superior improvements in blood sugar levels and significant weight loss, making it yet another breakthrough therapy. Clinical trials under the *SURPASS* program demonstrated that tirzepatide significantly lowered HbA1c levels and body weight more effectively than existing GLP-1 receptor agonists, including semaglutide. The popularity of Mounjaro has been growing rapidly since its approval, particularly because of its enhanced efficacy and the additional benefits of its dual receptor action. While Ozempic (semaglutide) remains a widely used and highly effective GLP-1 agonist, Mounjaro's ability to deliver better glycemic control and greater weight reduction is attracting considerable attention. However, both drugs have their unique advantages, and the choice between them often depends on individual patient needs and responses.

While Mounjaro shows exceptional promise and could potentially become more popular due to its superior weight loss results, Ozempic and Wegovy remain highly effective and widely used treatments. The competition among these medications is likely to drive further innovations and improvements in the treatment of diabetes and obesity, ultimately benefiting patients. In my professional opinion, what we are seeing is a growing knowledge base on weight loss and metabolic health, one that has taken off with breakneck speed. We are discovering more effective ways to aid weight loss and are positioning ourselves to understand our bodies in a deeper and more meaningful way. As I have already shared throughout the book, it is my belief that we can take this knowledge and exploit our natural resources to see similar results. Regardless if you take these medications or not, the reality is that we now have a means to successfully bridge the weight loss seen with GLP-1 optimization to sustainability and lifelong weight loss, which is something that has failed the vasty majority in the past. For this we can be grateful and look ahead to the future of weight management.

CHAPTER 5: STORIES OF TRANSFORMATION

The science behind semaglutides is undeniably compelling, but it's the real-life stories of transformation and, sometimes, disappointment that truly capture our imagination. After years of struggling with weight and its associated burdens, one discovers semaglutide therapy, with a promise of newfound freedom and vitality. The critical mistake that the vast majority make is not having a clearly defined semaglutide plan. One that accounts for the most common side effects and prepares the individual to conquer their post semaglutide lifestyle. The majority eagerly embrace this exciting new medication but lack the strategic understanding necessary to manage both the post fat loss response and the integration of lifestyle changes required to maintain their results. By holding this book, you are already a step ahead of these individuals. You will become equipped with the knowledge and strategies to ensure that your journey with semaglutide is not just a temporary fix but a lasting transformation.

I want you to feel excited and encouraged, however, it's important to acknowledge that not all stories of semaglutide use are destined for a happy ending. Consider the case of Laura, a 45-year-old professional who turned to semaglutide after battling obesity for most of her adult life. Initially, the results were promising; she experienced significant weight loss and felt more energetic than she had in years. But soon, Laura began to encounter severe gastrointestinal side effects, including persistent nausea and vomiting, which significantly impacted her daily life. Despite her weight loss, these side effects made it difficult for her to maintain her usual activities, and she found herself increasingly isolated and distressed. Additionally, Laura didn't have a comprehensive plan for life after semaglutide. Without proper guidance on how to maintain her weight loss through lifestyle interventions, she gradually regained the weight she had lost once she stopped the medication. There was also John, a 50-year-old businessman who had been struggling with his weight for years. After hearing about the success others had experienced with semaglutide, he decided to give it a try. Initially, John saw impressive results, losing over 30 pounds in a matter of months. He felt more energetic and confident, which positively impacted both his personal and professional life. Despite the initial weight loss, he found it challenging to maintain these results once he stopped taking semaglutide. Without a clear strategy for managing himself post-treatment, John gradually regained the weight. These very common stories underscore the necessity of a holistic approach to weight management—one that includes medical treatment, lifestyle changes, and ongoing support.

On the flip side, I've heard many wonderful stories, and I'm sure you have as well. Consider the story of Emily, a mother of two young children who had battled obesity for most of her adult life. She felt trapped in a cycle of frustration and despair, her energy levels plummeting, and her self-esteem eroding with each failed attempt at losing weight. Then, she discovered Ozempic. Within weeks, her life changed dramatically. Emily can feel optimistic regarding the future of her weight loss and health because she has a comprehensive and sensible post semaglutide game plan (this book). Her story of transformation isn't unique—it's happening repeatedly with these medications. However, when we revisit these individuals' journeys a year later, we often uncover a sad truth and a common thread of cautionary wisdom: keeping weight off is difficult, very difficult. We will go in depth into the mechanics of this reality in later chapters. Suffice to say, losing weight can feel like a downhill walk with semaglutide but you can be sure the path to keeping the weight off will offer a steep incline.

I wrote this book to provide that essential support and education, empowering you with the knowledge and tools necessary to thrive both on and off semaglutide. It's about understanding the science behind the medication, maximizing its benefits, and mitigating its potential drawbacks. Beyond medication, this book emphasizes developing a sustainable approach to weight management that includes healthy eating habits, regular exercise, and specific strategies for maintaining a healthy gut. My goal is to empower you to take charge of your health and well-being, enabling you to live a vibrant and fulfilling life long after your semaglutide journey is complete.

"I'm not telling you to take this [medication]. I'm telling you I did this for myself."
-Oprah Winfrey

Oprah Winfrey, a media icon and wellness advocate, has long been open about her struggles with weight. For years, she championed traditional methods like diet and exercise, believing that willpower alone could conquer the scale. Recently, Oprah shared a new chapter of her weight loss journey, one that involved a surprising twist: medication. Although she has not publicly disclosed the specific drug she used, it is widely speculated to be semaglutide and nearly guaranteed to be a drug that works as a GLP-1 agonist.

Her decision to turn to medication was not a sign of defeat but rather a testament to her evolving understanding of weight loss and the complex interplay of biology and behavior. "I had an awareness of [weight-loss] medications, but felt I had to prove I had the willpower to do it," Oprah confessed in an interview. "I now no longer feel that way." This shift in perspective reflects a growing recognition that weight loss is not solely a matter of willpower but a complex physiological and psychological challenge that often requires a multifaceted approach.

For Oprah, the medication acted as a catalyst, helping her break through a weight loss plateau and achieve her goals. It curbed her appetite, reduced cravings, and helped her feel satisfied with smaller portions. This newfound sense of control over her eating habits allowed her to focus on building healthier routines and making sustainable lifestyle changes. But Oprah's story is not just about the pounds lost; it's about the mental and emotional transformation that accompanied her weight loss journey. She speaks of feeling liberated from the shame and self-blame that often accompany weight struggles, embracing a more compassionate and accepting approach to her body. She talks about the newfound energy and vitality that have allowed her to engage more fully in her life, pursuing activities she once thought were out of reach.

Oprah's journey is a reminder that weight loss is not a linear path, but a winding road with twists, turns, and unexpected detours. It's a testament to the importance of self-compassion, resilience, and the willingness to explore all available tools and resources in the pursuit of health and well-being.

"I'm just ready to be on the field again"
-Ashley, mother of 3

Ashley was a high school athlete who "let herself go" after college and now finds it more difficult than ever to stay in shape with a full time job and three kids. She has always loved soccer and has a daughter who is following in her footsteps. Every time she watched her play from the sidelines, she imagined herself out there, wishing she had the confidence to coach the team or, at the very least, play with her daughter more often. Ashley felt that her weight was holding her back from being the mother she wanted to be and feared she wouldn't be able to keep up with the kids or be taken seriously by other parents. The thought of running up and down the field seemed like a distant dream.

Ashley had read a story about a woman who transformed her life with the help of semaglutide and decided to explore this option. Emily subsequently began her semaglutide journey. At first, the changes were small. She noticed she wasn't as hungry and had fewer cravings for the unhealthy snacks she used to rely on. Slowly but surely, the pounds started to come off. Each week, she felt a bit lighter and a lot more hopeful. The real turning point came when she played soccer with her daughter in the backyard and felt far less exhausted doing so. For the first time in years, she felt energized and capable.

Ashley's commitment paid off. By the end of summer, she had lost over 50 pounds and gained a newfound confidence. Compliments and inquiries were just a part of her daily life now. She has a post semaglutide plan in place and feels confident that she will be able to keep the weight off.

"Fasting + Ozempic/Wegovy + no tasty food near me"
-Elon Musk

Elon Musk, the visionary entrepreneur behind Tesla and SpaceX, is no stranger to pushing boundaries and embracing innovation. His relentless pursuit of progress extends beyond the realms of technology and into the sphere of personal health. Recently, Musk has openly acknowledged his use of Wegovy as part of his weight loss journey.

Musk shed a significant amount of fat, showcasing a leaner, more sculpted physique. The details of Musk's semaglutide experience remain somewhat shrouded in mystery. He has not publicly disclosed the exact dosage or duration of his treatment, nor has he elaborated on the specific ways in which the medication has impacted his appetite, cravings, or energy levels. However, his public acknowledgment of using Wegovy has sparked widespread interest and curiosity, further fueling the conversation about the role of GLP-1 receptor agonists in weight management.

However, Musk's story also serves as a cautionary tale. After initially losing weight with Wegovy, he reportedly gained some of it back, highlighting the challenges of maintaining weight loss after discontinuing the medication. This underscores the importance of transitioning from semaglutide to long-term lifestyle changes. Understanding this transition is crucial for sustaining weight loss and ensuring that the benefits of the medication are not short-lived but rather integrated into a comprehensive and lasting health strategy.

"I felt like myself again, the person I was before."

-Meredith, RN

Meredith, a busy nurse in her late thirties, had long struggled with her weight, despite her best efforts to maintain a healthy lifestyle. Years of yo-yo dieting, failed weight loss attempts and long shifts had left her feeling defeated and discouraged. When she discovered Ozempic, a flicker of hope ignited within her and she saw fantastic results. Within a couple short weeks, Meredith's appetite diminished significantly, her cravings subsided, and the scale began to reflect her progress. The weight loss was swift and steady, and with it came a renewed sense of energy, confidence, and vitality. "It was like a fog had lifted," she recalls.

But, alas, the journey was not without its challenges! The initial weeks on Ozempic brought bouts of the all familiar gastrointestinal side effects. Yet, for Meredith, these side effects paled in comparison to the newfound freedom and empowerment she was experiencing. As the pounds melted away, Meredith rediscovered the joy of movement, embracing activities she had once avoided due to self-consciousness. She found herself drawn to healthier foods, her cravings for sugary treats replaced by a newfound appreciation for the flavors and textures of whole, nutritious meals.

Meredith shared a different angle of her story that is important, openly discussing the hurdle of weaning off Ozempic. As we now know, maintaining her hard-earned progress without the medication's support would prove difficult but a necessary test of her new resolve for life. Her cravings returned and she was forced to confront the deeply ingrained habits that had contributed to her weight gain in the first place. Meredith has thus far succeeded in this battle, though it could easily have gone another direction. Her preparation for the difficulty surrounding stopping semaglutide could have been left much less to chance had she had a plan in place for the exit.

For those who find success with semaglutide, the journey extends beyond merely taking a medication; it's about embracing a holistic transformation. Lasting change requires more than just a prescription; it demands a commitment to lifestyle modifications, a willingness to explore new habits, and a dedication to self-care. These individuals approach semaglutide with curiosity and openness, eager to learn how the medication works in tandem with their bodies. They seek guidance and embrace a balanced lifestyle. They cultivate a mindful approach to eating, honoring their hunger and fullness cues, and savoring the pleasures of nourishing food.

For the others, the semaglutide journey often takes a different turn. They may experience initial success, shedding pounds and feeling a surge of energy. As time goes on, the medication's effects wane, and old habits resurface. Cravings return, willpower falters, and the scale creeps back up. These individuals often approach semaglutide with unrealistic expectations, viewing it as a quick fix or a substitute for healthy habits. They may neglect the importance of dietary changes and exercise, relying solely on the medication to do the heavy lifting. Lacking the support and guidance needed to navigate the challenges of weight loss, they feel isolated and discouraged. For these individuals, semaglutide becomes a temporary reprieve, a fleeting glimpse of a healthier future that quickly fades away. They may blame the medication for their lack of progress, failing to recognize that it's not a panacea but a tool that requires commitment and effort. Without integrating the necessary lifestyle changes and building a supportive network, the initial success achieved with semaglutide can be difficult to sustain, leading to disappointment and frustration.

The difference between successful and unsuccessful journeys with semaglutide lies not in the medication itself but in the individual's approach to it. Those who embrace semaglutide as part of a comprehensive lifestyle change program, who seek guidance and support, and who are willing to put in the work are more likely to achieve lasting success. Conversely, those who rely solely on the medication, neglecting the importance of healthy habits, are more likely to experience disappointment and frustration. This book aims to provide the support and education necessary to navigate the complexities of weight loss with semaglutide and to equip readers with the knowledge to maximize the benefits of the medication while integrating sustainable lifestyle changes that optimize your natural GLP-1 response for life.

With our time together thus far, we've explored the transformative potential and challenges of using semaglutide for weight management. We examined its history, starting with the development of early GLP-1 receptor agonists like exenatide and liraglutide, leading to the innovative semaglutide formulations found in Ozempic, Wegovy, and Rybelsus. We discussed real-life success stories, from Ashely to Oprah Winfrey, highlighting how semaglutide, when combined with lifestyle changes, can lead to significant weight loss and improved health. Conversely, we also addressed cautionary tales where individuals struggled due to lack of a comprehensive plan post-treatment, emphasizing the importance of integrating medication with holistic lifestyle changes for sustained results. Finally, we underscored the necessity of education, support, and realistic expectations in maximizing the benefits of semaglutide, transforming it from a temporary aid into a long-term ally in achieving health and wellness.

Next, I will guide you on an exploration of the science behind GLP-1 and semaglutide. Whether you're a medical professional, a science enthusiast, or simply someone who wants a deeper understanding of how these medications work, this section aims to provide comprehensive insights.

In this section, we will delve into the biochemical foundations of GLP-1. We will explore how GLP-1 functions in our daily lives, influencing processes like insulin secretion, glucagon suppression, and gastric emptying, and how these mechanisms contribute to its effectiveness in managing type 2 diabetes and obesity. We will also take a closer look at semaglutide, examining its pharmacodynamics, and pharmacokinetics. You'll learn how semaglutide mimics the action of natural GLP-1 to enhance insulin secretion, reduce appetite, and promote weight loss. Detailed explanations will be provided on its dosing regimens, including the standard protocols and the emerging concept of microdosing, which holds promise for optimizing benefits while broadening patient capture and medication use in society. We will also be discussing, at length, the potential adverse effects associated with semaglutide use. From common issues like nausea and gastrointestinal discomfort to more serious concerns like pancreatitis and thyroid tumors, we will cover the spectrum of possible reactions and the clinical strategies used to manage them.

This deep dive is designed for those who crave a detailed understanding of the science behind semaglutide. However, if you find that this level of detail exceeds your desire for knowledge, feel free to skip ahead. The subsequent sections offer valuable insights and practical advice for integrating semaglutide into a holistic approach to health and weight management. Prepare to embark on a scientific journey that reveals the intricate workings of GLP-1 and semaglutide, I hope you find it a rich perspective on these therapies.

SECTION II: GLP-1 IN YOUR BODY (PHYSIOLOGY)

CHAPTER 6: THE DAILY ROLE OF GLP-1

Before embarking on this book, I sought to understand the minute-to-minute, hour-to-hour impact of GLP-1 on health. My goal was to piece together why semaglutide works so effectively and what might be malfunctioning in the GLP-1 response of those struggling with weight issues.

GLP-1 is a crucial hormone in the regulation of metabolism, playing an integral role in maintaining health. This hormone is produced by L-cells in the distal ileum and colon, and its secretion is stimulated by nutrient intake. Upon release, GLP-1 engages in a coordinated symphony of actions affecting several key organs and systems to regulate blood sugar levels and appetite.

During meals, GLP-1 gets to work. As you eat breakfast, GLP-1 helps your brain recognize fullness, curbing the urge to overeat. This recognition of fullness involves several specific brain centers that play crucial roles in appetite regulation and energy balance. Specifically within the hypothalamus, the arcuate nucleus (ARC) is particularly significant. The ARC contains two types of neurons: the orexigenic neurons that stimulate appetite and the anorexigenic neurons that suppress it. GLP-1 receptors in the ARC help modulate these neurons, reducing hunger signals and promoting feelings of satiety. Another important area is the brainstem, specifically the nucleus tractus solitarius (NTS). The NTS receives direct signals from the gastrointestinal tract via the vagus nerve, relaying information about nutrient intake and energy status to higher brain centers. GLP-1 released from the gut can act on the NTS, enhancing its ability to signal fullness to the brain. This action helps to ensure that the body appropriately regulates food intake based on the amount of food consumed. Additionally, the ventromedial hypothalamus (VMH) and the dorsomedial hypothalamus (DMH) also play roles in mediating the effects of GLP-1. These areas are involved in integrating metabolic signals and regulating energy expenditure. The activation of GLP-1 receptors in these regions contributes to the overall sensation of fullness and helps balance energy intake and expenditure. The insular cortex is another brain region implicated in the process. It is involved in the subjective experience of hunger and satiety. This is an important one and quelling this subjective response can have obvious positive consequences.

GLP-1 plays an intricate role in regulating insulin secretion and gastrointestinal activity, which in turn influences blood sugar levels and satiety. The initial release of GLP-1 is highly sensitive to the size and composition of the meal. For example, a light lunch triggers a moderate release of GLP-1, while a more substantial dinner prompts a more significant response. This ensures a proportional and appropriate physiological reaction to varying nutrient loads.

When GLP-1 is released, it enhances the glucose-dependent secretion of insulin from the pancreatic beta cells. This mechanism is crucial because it ensures that insulin is secreted in response to elevated blood glucose levels, thereby maintaining stable blood sugar levels. This action helps prevent hyperglycemia, a condition characterized by excessive glucose in the bloodstream, which is particularly important for individuals with type 2 diabetes. Simultaneously, GLP-1 inhibits the secretion of glucagon from the pancreatic alpha cells. Glucagon is a hormone that stimulates the liver to convert stored glycogen into glucose, which is then released into the bloodstream. By suppressing glucagon secretion, GLP-1 reduces the liver's glucose output. This inhibition is crucial after meals when blood glucose levels are already elevated due to nutrient intake. By moderating the release of glucose from the liver, GLP-1 helps prevent postprandial hyperglycemia (high blood sugar levels following a meal).

GLP-1 also enhances insulin sensitivity in the liver. When it stimulates the release of insulin from the pancreatic beta cells, insulin then acts on the liver to promote glucose uptake and storage as glycogen. Glycogen serves as a storage form of glucose, which can be mobilized during periods of fasting or increased energy demand. Enhanced glycogen synthesis ensures that glucose is effectively stored for future use, contributing to overall metabolic stability. Overall, this process helps lower blood glucose levels.

GLP-1 also influences lipid metabolism in the liver. It has been shown to reduce hepatic steatosis (fat accumulation in the liver), which is beneficial for preventing non-alcoholic fatty liver disease (NAFLD). This is another key point of contribution for semaglutides, as fatty liver is reaching epidemic proportions. By promoting fat oxidation and reducing the synthesis of new fats, GLP-1 helps maintain healthier liver function, a crucial aspect of the poor metabolic health we are seeing in today's world.

As mentioned, upon ingestion of food, GLP-1 is secreted by the L-cells in the ileum and colon. One of its primary effects is to slow gastric emptying, a process regulated by several mechanisms. When GLP-1 binds to its receptors in the stomach and small intestine, it modulates the activity of the enteric nervous system and the central nervous system, which together coordinate digestive motility. This interaction leads to a reduction in the rate at which the stomach contents are transferred to the duodenum, the first part of the small intestine. The stomach's pyloric sphincter, which regulates the passage of stomach contents into the duodenum, is influenced by GLP-1. The hormone's action on this sphincter slows its opening, thus delaying gastric emptying. Additionally, the interaction with the enteric nervous system helps coordinate muscle contractions in the gastrointestinal tract to slow the transit time of food.

The slowing of gastric emptying has several metabolic benefits. It prolongs the period during which nutrients are absorbed in the small intestine. By doing so, it allows for a more gradual absorption of glucose, which helps to prevent rapid spikes in blood glucose levels after a meal. This is particularly beneficial for individuals with diabetes, as it aids in maintaining more stable blood sugar levels, reducing the risk of hyperglycemia. By extending the duration of nutrient absorption, GLP-1 enhances the feeling of fullness or satiety that we learned about in the brain. Furthermore, this mechanism plays a role in the overall energy balance and metabolic health of the body. By slowing the digestive process, GLP-1 ensures that nutrients are utilized more effectively, supporting the body's metabolic needs without overwhelming the system with rapid influxes of glucose and other nutrients. This sophisticated interplay underscores the hormone's critical function in metabolic regulation and its potential as a therapeutic target.

As evening approaches, the physiological role of GLP-1 undergoes a significant shift to support the body's transition into the fasting state and to prepare for nighttime rest. This transition involves intricate interactions with multiple organs and regulatory systems, ensuring energy homeostasis and metabolic balance throughout the night. As GLP-1 activity decreases in the evening, one of its critical roles is to signal the liver to manage glucose levels during the overnight fasting period. As food intake ceases in the evening, GLP-1's effect on insulin diminishes, and glucagon levels rise. This rise in glucagon prompts the liver to release stored glucose through glycogenolysis and gluconeogenesis, ensuring a steady supply of glucose to maintain blood sugar levels and provide necessary cellular energy throughout the night.

GLP-1 also affects lipid metabolism and fat storage during the night by regulating the balance between lipogenesis (fat storage) and lipolysis (fat breakdown). This balance is essential for preventing excessive fat accumulation, particularly in the liver, which is crucial for avoiding fatty liver disease, high triglycerides and a cholesterol panel that makes your primary care provider sweat.

GLP-1 also communicates with the central nervous system, particularly influencing areas of the brain involved in relaxation and sleep regulation. Back in the hypothalamus, GLP-1 contributes to the modulation of circadian rhythms and promotes the transition from wakefulness to sleep. It helps regulate the release of neurotransmitters that induce relaxation and sleep, such as gamma-aminobutyric acid (GABA) and melatonin. This interaction ensures that the body prepares adequately for restful sleep, which we know is absolutely critical to overall health.

While the digestive system slows down at night, GLP-1 still influences gastrointestinal function to a certain extent. It ensures that any residual food in the stomach and intestines is processed efficiently and that gastric emptying is appropriately modulated. This continued modulation helps maintain satiety, preventing nighttime hunger and unnecessary caloric intake that could disrupt metabolic balance.

When writing this book, I was quite impressed with the extensive role that GLP-1 plays in metabolic health. Armed with this knowledge, suddenly, semaglutides made a whole lot of sense. Simply imagine GLP-1 functioning at only 90% capacity, how much would your appetite change, your blood glucose de-regulate and your digestion shift toward non-optimal? Once I had studied this system fully and understood all the hats that GLP-1 wears in our metabolic play, it was extremely clear to me just how optimizing function of this hormone could truly transform metabolic health.

It is important to understand that the GLP-1 response and function operate on a spectrum, rather than in a binary on/off manner. This means it is entirely possible to have partial function, a less robust response, or receptors that are not functioning optimally. Think of the GLP-1 receptor as a sophisticated thermostat—it's not just an on/off switch but a device capable of fine-tuning your body's metabolic processes. As you are now aware, this receptor is found in various tissues throughout your body, which explains how GLP-1 can affect multiple systems. The health and response of these receptors can vary significantly within each tissue.

Semaglutide essentially enhances this thermostat's ability to precisely control your body's energy balance. It doesn't just turn the heat up or down; it optimizes the temperature to suit your individual needs. This fine-tuning ability is where the concept of "partial agonism" comes into play. Semaglutide can partially activate the GLP-1 receptors, providing a nuanced and tailored response that can improve metabolic outcomes. This sophisticated mechanism allows for better management.

Secondary to this, some people may be more sensitive to semaglutide, while others may require a higher dose to achieve the same effect. By tailoring the treatment to your individual needs, you can maximize the benefits of GLP-1 receptor agonism while minimizing potential side effects.

When using semaglutide, it is administered in doses much higher than what the body naturally produces. This is referred to as a "supraphysiologic" dose. These elevated levels of GLP-1 disrupt the natural rhythm of the hormone. While this disruption is intentional and mostly beneficial in the short term, enhancing the therapeutic effects of GLP-1, it raises questions about potential long-term consequences. One concern is the impact on the body's natural ability to produce and regulate GLP-1 after discontinuing semaglutide. Similar to how a bodybuilder might struggle to produce natural testosterone after prolonged use of exogenous steroids, there is concern about the body's ability to produce GLP-1 post-semaglutide use. Chronic exposure to high levels of exogenous GLP-1 from medications like semaglutide may lead to a downregulation of GLP-1 receptors, making the body less responsive to the hormone's signals. This receptor downregulation could impair the body's natural ability to regulate appetite and blood sugar levels, potentially leading to a rebound effect when the medication is stopped.

Another concern is the impact on the circadian rhythm itself. The body's natural rhythms are finely tuned, and disrupting them can have cascading effects on various physiological processes. Chronic disruption of the GLP-1 rhythm may lead to alterations in other hormonal rhythms, such as cortisol, melatonin, and growth hormone, potentially impacting sleep, stress response, and overall health. Furthermore, the long-term effects of supraphysiologic

GLP-1 levels on the pancreas and other organs are still under investigation. While GLP-1 receptor agonists have been shown to be safe and effective in the short term, their long-term impact on pancreatic beta-cell function, insulin sensitivity, and the risk of pancreatitis is not yet fully understood.

Given the advent of newer medications with multiple receptor effects, such as Mounjaro, which combines GLP-1 and GIP agonism, it is important to discuss future modalities in relation to the content of this book. Gastric Inhibitory Polypeptide (GIP) is another incretin hormone that plays a significant role in metabolic regulation, working synergistically with GLP-1. Research into GIP is revealing its potential to complement GLP-1 therapies, and combining GLP-1 and GIP receptor agonists may result in enhanced therapeutic effects.

The exploration of hunger hormones extends beyond GLP-1 and GIP. Emerging therapies are focusing on other hormones such as ghrelin, peptide YY (PYY), and others that regulate appetite and energy homeostasis. These future modalities aim to provide a comprehensive approach to appetite control and weight management. However, it is important to understand that the strategies detailed in this book will only become more powerful as new medications evolve. The information presented here will not become obsolete, you are learning to optimize all hunger hormones. Read on with confidence, knowing that the principles within this book are foundational and will remain relevant as medical science progresses.

CHAPTER 7: GLP-1 RESPONDS TO NATURE

GLP-1 has a rhythm, a natural ebb and flow that aligns with the tides of daily life and the changing seasons. This rhythmic nature of GLP-1 is crucial because it interacts intricately with the body's various biological clocks. Our bodies operate within a complex framework of rhythms, which govern daily physiological processes, as well as weekly and seasonal rhythms that affect everything from mood to metabolism.

The 24-hour circadian rhythm is a cornerstone of human physiology, orchestrating a variety of biological processes to align with the environmental day-night cycle. Central to this rhythm is the suprachiasmatic nucleus (SCN) in the hypothalamus, which functions as the master clock. The SCN receives direct input from the retina via the retinohypothalamic tract, enabling it to synchronize the internal clock with external light-dark cycles. This synchronization ensures a coherent rhythmic pattern across different physiological systems, coordinating the activity of peripheral clocks found in various tissues and organs. The circadian rhythm profoundly impacts the sleep-wake cycle. The SCN signals the release of hormones and neurotransmitters that regulate alertness and sleepiness. During the day, exposure to light inhibits melatonin production and promotes wakefulness. As evening approaches and light decreases, melatonin production ramps up, preparing the body for sleep. This rhythmic release of hormones and the corresponding physiological changes are essential for maintaining a consistent sleep schedule and overall health.

As I just alluded to, regulation of hormonal secretion is a critical component of the circadian rhythm. Cortisol, often referred to as the "stress hormone," follows a diurnal pattern, peaking in the early morning around 8 AM and gradually declining throughout the day to its lowest levels in the late evening. This pattern supports metabolism, immune response, and stress management. As it happens, this pattern is completely dysregulated in today's overly stressed society. Conversely, melatonin, the hormone responsible for promoting sleep, is secreted by the pineal gland with levels rising in the evening as darkness falls, peaking in the middle of the night around 2-4 AM, and tapering off by morning. Melatonin's release is pivotal for regulating the sleep-wake cycle and promoting restful sleep. Probably unsurprisingly, millions of individuals suffer from very poor melatonin cycling.

Growth hormone, which is crucial for growth, cell repair, and metabolism, also follows a circadian pattern. Its secretion predominantly occurs during deep sleep stages, especially in the first half of the night. This nocturnal release supports bodily repair and growth processes. Poor cortisol cycling + dysregulated melatonin patterning = low quality sleep and terrible growth hormone levels = waning overall health. Are you starting to see the patterns connecting here?

In addition to hormonal regulation, the circadian rhythm influences body temperature, digestion, and cardiovascular function. Body temperature typically peaks in the late afternoon and early evening and reaches its lowest point in the early morning hours, just before waking. Digestive processes are also regulated, with enzyme activity and nutrient absorption being optimized during the day when food intake is expected. Similarly, cardiovascular function varies throughout the day, with blood pressure and heart rate generally being higher during waking hours and lower during sleep, reflecting the body's rest and activity cycles.

The synchronization of these physiological processes with the 24-hour day-night cycle is vital for optimal functioning and health. Disruptions to the circadian rhythm, such as those caused by shift work, travel across time zones, or exposure to artificial light at night, can lead to various health issues, including sleep disorders, metabolic syndrome, cardiovascular diseases, and mood disorders. Understanding the 24-hour circadian rhythm provides insight into how our bodies maintain balance and function effectively. This knowledge underscores the importance of aligning our lifestyles with natural rhythms to promote health and well-being. By recognizing the critical role of the circadian clock, we can better appreciate the need for consistent sleep patterns, regular exposure to natural light, and the timing of meals and activities to support our internal biological rhythms.

The human body also follows a less well-known but equally significant weekly cycle, known as the "circaseptan" rhythm. This seven-day biological rhythm influences various physiological and behavioral processes, reflecting an intrinsic temporal organization that aligns with the seven-day week, even in the absence of external cues.

Research suggests that this weekly rhythm may have evolutionary roots, possibly linked to social and environmental factors. For instance, early human societies may have adopted a seven-day cycle due to the lunar calendar or other natural cycles, and this external structure could have become internalized over generations. One of the key aspects of the circaseptan rhythm is its impact on the immune system. Studies have shown that certain immune functions, such as the production of antibodies and the activity of natural killer cells, fluctuate on a weekly basis. For example, patients recovering from surgery or managing chronic illnesses often exhibit cyclical patterns in their symptoms, with some days showing significant improvement while others may see a decline. This periodicity suggests an underlying biological rhythm that could influence recovery and disease progression.

Cardiovascular health is also influenced by the weekly cycle. Research indicates that the risk of heart attacks and strokes varies throughout the week, with higher incidences reported on certain days. This pattern might be associated with the stress of returning to work after the weekend or other lifestyle factors, but it also points to an intrinsic weekly rhythm that affects cardiovascular function.

Hormones like cortisol and serotonin exhibit weekly fluctuations. These hormonal rhythms may contribute to variations in energy levels, mood, and overall well-being throughout the week. For instance, some people might experience a peak in energy and mood mid-week, while others feel more fatigued and stressed at the beginning or end of the week.

Sleep patterns and activity levels also reflect a weekly rhythm. Many individuals tend to get more sleep on weekends, using this time to recover from the sleep debt accumulated during the workweek. This cycle of sleep deprivation and catch-up can impact overall sleep quality and health. Additionally, physical activity levels often vary, with people being more active on weekends due to more free time and recreational opportunities. Understanding the weekly rhythm's influence on health can have practical applications in medicine and wellness. For example, recognizing these patterns can help optimize the timing of medication administration, known as chronotherapy, to align with the body's natural rhythms for better efficacy and reduced side effects. It can also inform work schedules and stress management strategies to enhance productivity and well-being.

Human biology is deeply influenced by seasonal rhythms, which are cyclic changes occurring throughout the year in response to variations in daylight, temperature, and other environmental factors. These rhythms, known as circannual rhythms, affect numerous physiological and behavioral processes, including hormonal cycles, immune function, metabolism, and mood.

There is a seasonal surge in GLP-1 that coincides with trends in weight loss and metabolic health improvements often observed during summer. Studies indicate that individuals tend to lose weight more easily and maintain better blood sugar control in the summer months. While it is challenging to establish a direct causal relationship, the correlation between higher GLP-1 levels and improved metabolic outcomes is intriguing and significant. The potential implications of this connection are vast. Assuming the significance of summer changes are secondary to increased sunlight, we can assume that GLP-1 is affected by sunlight. If this does indeed boost GLP-1 levels, it offers a simple and accessible way to improve metabolic health and support weight loss efforts.

Seasonal changes significantly impact hormonal secretion. For instance, melatonin is highly sensitive to variations in daylight. During the shorter days of winter, melatonin production increases, resulting in longer periods of elevated melatonin levels at night. This increase can influence sleep patterns and contribute to the winter blues or seasonal affective disorder (SAD). Conversely, during the longer days of summer, melatonin levels decrease, supporting shorter and more restful sleep periods. Cortisol levels tend to be higher in the winter, potentially due to increased physical and psychological stressors, such as colder temperatures and less daylight. These elevated cortisol levels can impact immune function, metabolism, and mood.

Speaking of immune function, this system exhibits seasonal variability as well. Studies have shown that immune cell activity fluctuates with the seasons, potentially due to changes in vitamin D levels from sunlight exposure. In the summer, higher levels of sunlight lead to increased production of vitamin D, which plays a crucial role in enhancing immune response. Conversely, during the winter months, reduced sunlight exposure can lead to lower vitamin D levels, potentially weakening the immune system and increasing susceptibility to infections.

Metabolic processes and energy balance are also influenced by seasonal rhythms. In colder months, the body tends to increase energy expenditure to maintain core temperature, potentially leading to increased appetite and caloric intake. This physiological response can result in weight gain during the winter. Conversely, during the warmer months, there is often a natural decrease in appetite and an increase in physical activity, promoting weight loss and improved metabolic health. Seasonal changes in daylight and temperature also significantly impact mood and behavior. The prevalence of mood disorders, such as seasonal affective disorder (SAD), increases during the winter months when daylight is scarce. Reduced sunlight exposure can lower serotonin levels in the brain, contributing to feelings of depression and lethargy. In contrast, increased sunlight during the summer boosts serotonin production, enhancing mood and energy levels.

Seasonal variations also affect cardiovascular health. Research indicates that blood pressure and cholesterol levels tend to be higher in the winter months for all of the reasons previously stated. These factors can elevate the risk of cardiovascular events, such as heart attacks and strokes, during colder months. Conversely, improved cardiovascular function is often observed in the summer.

Building a long-term plan for weight loss involving semaglutide is a complex endeavor, largely due to the intricate interplay between the body's various biological rhythms and the role of GLP-1 within these cycles. Each rhythm affects GLP-1 secretion and action, adding layers of complexity to the management of metabolic health and weight.

The 24-hour circadian rhythm significantly influences GLP-1 levels. GLP-1 secretion is synchronized with meal times, peaking in response to food intake. Disruptions to the circadian rhythm can lead to misalignment in GLP-1 secretion. Weekly rhythms cause variations in stress and physical activity levels throughout the week that can alter insulin sensitivity and appetite. During the winter months, reduced sunlight exposure can disrupt circadian rhythms, lower vitamin D levels, and decrease physical activity, all of which can lead to a decline in GLP-1 levels. The shift towards heavier, less fiber-rich foods in colder months can further diminish GLP-1 secretion, challenging efforts to maintain weight loss and metabolic health. This underscores the importance of maintaining a consistent schedule, sleeping well, getting outdoors often, feeling the morning sun on your skin and putting your feet on the ground. We are looking to optimize the efficacy of semaglutide and natural GLP-1.

Considering both established knowledge and theoretical implications, the long-term effects of chronic GLP-1 agonist use necessitate careful evaluation and management. Supraphysiologic doses of semaglutide significantly elevate the levels of this hormone in the body, which can disrupt natural hormonal rhythms. Can these high levels of exogenous hormone cause further disruption in overweight individual's biological rhythms?

As we discussed previously, chronic exposure to high levels of exogenous GLP-1 can lead to receptor downregulation. This is a well-documented phenomenon in endocrinology, where receptors become desensitized due to persistent stimulation. Studies have shown that prolonged exposure to GLP-1 receptor agonists can result in a decreased number of available receptors, potentially reducing the body's responsiveness to both endogenous and exogenous GLP-1. This downregulation poses a risk when discontinuing GLP-1 therapy, as the reduced receptor sensitivity could impair the body's natural ability to regulate blood glucose levels and appetite, leading to potential rebound weight gain and metabolic dysregulation.

Another concern is the potential impact on the body's natural production of GLP-1. The endocrine system often operates on feedback mechanisms, where the presence of an exogenous hormone can signal the body to reduce its endogenous production. With prolonged GLP-1 agonist use, there is a theoretical risk that the L-cells in the intestines may decrease their natural secretion of GLP-1. This could lead to a dependency on the medication for maintaining metabolic control, making it challenging to discontinue therapy without adverse effects.

Circling back around to biological rhythms, one theoretical approach to mitigate these risks involves mimicking the body's natural fluctuations in GLP-1 levels. By adjusting the dosing regimen to align more closely with physiological rhythms, it might be possible to maintain therapeutic benefits while reducing the risk of receptor downregulation and preserving endogenous GLP-1 production. For example, intermittent dosing schedules or tapering strategies could help the body adapt to lower levels of exogenous GLP-1 gradually, promoting a more natural regulatory environment.

While I present some theories here, what is clear is that aligning yourself with natural rhythms of the body will optimize all hormone production, including optimized function of GLP-1, and will expand your health repertoire. Adapting yourself to the rigid structure of our natural rhythms is one of the critical components of building a post semaglutide lifestyle that allows for sustainable weight loss.

CHAPTER 8: GLP-1 FUNCTION IN THIN PEOPLE

While semaglutide has shown remarkable promise in treating type 2 diabetes and obesity, the question of whether everyone should seek to increase GLP-1 activation is more nuanced. Should we all be trying to increase our natural GLP-1 response? Do people who never struggle with weight loss naturally have higher GLP-1 levels, more receptors, or both?

Research indicates that thinner, healthier individuals often exhibit higher levels of naturally produced GLP-1 compared to those with obesity or metabolic disorders. This finding is particularly evident in populations with lower rates of type 2 diabetes, such as those adhering to traditional cultural patterns characterized by diets rich in whole foods, regular and strenuous physical activity, and healthier environmental lifestyles. These observations suggest that lifestyle plays a significant role in modulating GLP-1 activity and may contribute to the lower prevalence of metabolic disorders in these populations.

Traditional diets typically emphasize whole, unprocessed foods, which are rich in fiber, vitamins, and minerals. Foods like vegetables, fruits, legumes, nuts, and whole grains are staples in these diets. High-fiber foods, in particular, are known to stimulate GLP-1 secretion. Fiber is fermented by gut microbiota into short-chain fatty acids, which in turn promote GLP-1 release from L-cells in the intestine. Additionally, whole foods provide essential nutrients that support overall metabolic health and enhance the body's natural GLP-1 response.

Physical activity is another crucial factor influencing GLP-1 levels. Regular exercise has been shown to enhance GLP-1 secretion and improve insulin sensitivity . Physical activity increases the expression of GLP-1 receptors and promotes the release of the hormone during and after exercise. Populations with active lifestyles, whether through manual labor, traditional farming, or regular exercise routines, tend to maintain healthier body weights and better metabolic profiles. This regular, strenuous physical activity contributes to the robust GLP-1 response observed in these populations.

Healthier environmental lifestyles encompass various factors, including reduced exposure to environmental toxins, lower stress levels, and better sleep quality. Traditional lifestyles often involve more time spent outdoors, leading to increased sunlight exposure, which helps regulate circadian rhythms and hormonal balance, including GLP-1 secretion. Reduced exposure to pollutants and endocrine-disrupting chemicals, commonly found in industrialized environments, also supports healthier metabolic function . Furthermore, lower stress levels and better sleep quality, often associated with less hectic and more community-oriented lifestyles, contribute to overall hormonal balance and improved GLP-1 activity.

Cultural practices and social structures play a significant role in promoting healthy behaviors that enhance GLP-1 levels. Traditional societies often emphasize communal eating, meal preparation, and physical activity, which foster healthier dietary habits and more consistent physical exercise routines. These cultural practices not only support better nutrition and fitness but also promote mental well-being and stress reduction, further contributing to healthier metabolic profiles .

The correlation between traditional lifestyles and healthier GLP-1 levels suggests that modern health interventions can benefit from integrating these cultural practices. Encouraging diets rich in whole foods, promoting regular physical activity, and fostering community-based health initiatives can help improve GLP-1 response and overall metabolic health. Understanding the mechanisms behind these cultural patterns provides valuable insights for designing effective public health strategies and personalized treatments for metabolic disorders.

There is a bit of a chicken or egg conundrum at play here; do healthy people enhance their GLP-1 responses better than the unhealthy, or do healthy people naturally have higher GLP-1 levels which render them more capable of making healthier lifestyle choices? Unfortunately, we don't know, and it's a complex issue.

GLP-1's role in metabolic health is significant but interwoven with other elements such as genetics, gut microbiota, and environmental influences. For instance, genetic variations can affect GLP-1 receptor expression and function, potentially influencing an individual's response to GLP-1. Similarly, the gut microbiota can modulate GLP-1 secretion by fermenting dietary fibers into short-chain fatty acids, which then stimulate GLP-1 release. These factors add additional layers of complexity to understanding how GLP-1 interacts with other elements of metabolic regulation.

However, the interplay between GLP-1 and these factors can be bidirectional. Enhanced GLP-1 activity can improve insulin sensitivity, promote satiety, and reduce inflammation, which in turn can positively influence gut microbiota composition, genetic expression, and environmental resilience. This suggests that optimizing GLP-1 response through lifestyle changes and potentially pharmacological interventions like semaglutide could create a positive feedback loop, enhancing overall metabolic health.

As we transition from discussing the natural GLP-1 response in healthier individuals, it is crucial to understand the primary physiological effects of semaglutide. Semaglutide is designed to mimic the natural hormone's actions, significantly impacting three primary mechanisms: appetite suppression, blood glucose regulation and the slowing of digestive processes. For the next few chapters, we will delve into how semaglutide modulates these key processes, thereby improving metabolic health and supporting effective weight management. This exploration will provide a comprehensive understanding of how semaglutide works within the body to achieve its remarkable clinical outcomes.

CHAPTER 9: POWERFUL APPETITE SUPPRESSION

To appreciate how semaglutide modulates appetite, it's important to first understand the normal physiological processes that regulate hunger and satiety. The regulation of hunger and satiety involves a complex interplay between the digestive system, endocrine signals, and neural pathways, ensuring that energy intake matches the body's needs.

The sensation of hunger is primarily driven by the hormone ghrelin, often referred to as the "hunger hormone." Ghrelin is produced by the stomach and its levels rise before meals, signaling the brain to stimulate appetite. This process begins when the stomach is empty, causing ghrelin levels to increase and send signals to the hypothalamus. Ghrelin binds to receptors here, promoting the sensation of hunger and motivating food intake. The hypothalamus integrates these signals with other inputs, such as blood glucose levels, to regulate energy intake. Low blood glucose levels also stimulate hunger, signaling the need for energy replenishment. This intricate system ensures that the body seeks food when energy stores are low.

Satiety, the feeling of fullness that stops us from eating, involves several hormones and neural signals. One of the key players in this process is GLP-1, which helps to promote a feeling of fullness and a reduction in the speed at which nutrients enter the bloodstream. Other important satiety hormones include peptide YY (PYY) and cholecystokinin (CCK). PYY is secreted by the ileum and colon in response to food intake, especially protein and fat, and works to reduce appetite. CCK is released from the small intestine and stimulates the digestion of fat and protein while also sending signals to the brain to induce satiety.

The brainstem and the hypothalamus play critical roles in processing these satiety signals. When food enters the stomach and intestines, these organs send neural signals through the vagus nerve to the brainstem, which then communicates with the hypothalamus to signal fullness. This complex signaling network ensures that once enough food has been consumed, the drive to eat diminishes.

The balance between hunger and satiety signals maintains energy homeostasis. After eating, ghrelin levels fall, and satiety hormones like GLP-1, PYY, and CCK rise, reducing appetite and promoting feelings of fullness. This balance prevents overeating and helps regulate body weight. However, in individuals with obesity or metabolic disorders, this regulatory system can become disrupted. Hormonal imbalances, such as leptin resistance or chronic high levels of ghrelin, can impair the normal response to hunger and satiety signals, leading to overeating and weight gain.

This disruption highlights the potential therapeutic role of medications like semaglutide, which can help restore the balance by enhancing satiety signals and reducing hunger. Imagine a volume knob on your appetite, with semaglutide effectively turning it down, transforming the once-deafening roar of hunger into a mere whisper. Semaglutide gently nudges your body's natural satiety signals, making it easier to heed your body's cues and stop eating when you're physiologically satisfied.

For some individuals, semaglutide may correct an underlying physiologic imbalance, restoring their appetite to a more normal level. These people might have hormonal imbalances that amplify hunger signals, making it difficult to maintain a healthy weight. Semaglutide can help modulate these signals, reducing the intensity of hunger and aiding in weight management. For others, semaglutide helps overcome environmental and behavioral factors that have led to unhealthy eating patterns. With cheap, low quality, easily accessible high-calorie foods available everywhere, many people struggle with overeating. Semaglutide makes it easier to resist overeating and to choose healthier foods. In both scenarios, the goal is to achieve a sustainable and healthy weight through a combination of medication and lifestyle changes. Semaglutide facilitates this process by making it easier to adhere to a balanced regimen of lifestyle modifications, ultimately leading to improved metabolic health and well-being.

The feeling of contentment with smaller portions is a key aspect of semaglutide's impact on appetite. This effect is not about feeling deprived or restricted but rather experiencing a genuine sense of satisfaction with less food. It leads to a natural reduction in calorie intake without the need for strict portion control or calorie counting. This principle, often mastered through years of disciplined eating, is offered more effortlessly to those with an optimized GLP-1 response.

Take the people of Okinawa, Japan, for example. Known for their enduring health and low prevalence of obesity, they practice "hara hachi bu," a centuries-old cultural norm that means "eating until you are 80% full." This profound concept encourages mindful eating and promotes long-term health by establishing a habit of eating to basic satisfaction. It involves stopping before feeling completely stuffed, leaving a little room in the stomach, and avoiding the discomfort of overeating. Okinawans, who have one of the highest life expectancies in the world, attribute their longevity in part to this practice. They believe that eating until 80% full helps maintain a healthy weight, improve digestion, boost energy levels, and reduce the risk of chronic diseases. Scientific studies support the benefits of such mindful eating practices, showing that they can lead to lower caloric intake and improved metabolic health. Semaglutide users can achieve similar benefits as those seen in the Okinawan practice, by being given an easier method toward "hara hachi bu."

The question of whether individuals with obesity inherently have greater appetites is complex, with no straightforward answer. While it may seem intuitive to assume that overweight individuals consume more calories simply due to larger appetites, the reality is far more nuanced.

The perception of hunger and satiety is highly individualized, influenced by a person's unique physiologic, psychologic, and environmental contexts. This diversity means that addressing obesity requires personalized approaches that consider the multifaceted nature of appetite regulation and energy balance. Some studies have suggested that individuals with obesity may have a blunted response to satiety signals. This could be due to a variety of factors, including genetic predisposition, alterations in gut microbiota, or even psychologic factors like emotional eating patterns. Moreover, appetite is not solely determined by biologic factors. Environmental and behavioral factors also play a significant role. Emotional eating patterns and habits formed around food can override physiologic hunger signals, leading to overconsumption. In helping absolutely nothing but the company's bottom line, food is even engineered these days to ensure that you overeat it.

For some individuals, hormonal imbalances such as leptin resistance or elevated ghrelin levels contribute to increased hunger and cravings. Leptin normally signals satiety to the brain, but in leptin resistance, this signaling is impaired, leading to persistent hunger despite adequate or excess energy stores. Similarly, elevated ghrelin levels can exacerbate feelings of hunger and contribute to overeating. These hormonal disruptions can create a vicious cycle of overeating and weight gain, making it difficult for individuals to feel full and satisfied. This cycle perpetuates itself, as the body's regulatory mechanisms for hunger and satiety are compromised. However, it is important to note that not everyone with obesity experiences heightened appetite.

Metabolic adaptations in response to weight gain significantly alter energy expenditure and storage, adding complexity to the relationship between appetite and obesity. When an individual gains weight, especially through increased fat mass, the body undergoes a series of metabolic changes aimed at maintaining energy balance. These adaptations include alterations in basal metabolic rate (BMR), thermogenesis, and nutrient partitioning.

Basal metabolic rate, the amount of energy expended at rest, can increase with weight gain due to the higher energy requirements of maintaining a larger body mass. However, this increase is not always proportional to the weight gained. In some cases, the body becomes more efficient at conserving energy, reducing BMR relative to what would be expected based on body size alone. This efficiency is a survival mechanism, keeping one alive in the ice age. However, it is a rather large burden in the era of mocha frappes and potato chips. This adaptation prevents energy depletion overall, whether you are in a time of scarcity (incredibly rare) or abundance (incredibly common).

Thermogenesis, the process of heat production in the body, is another area affected by weight gain. Adaptive thermogenesis can occur, where the body adjusts its energy expenditure in response to changes in diet and energy balance. For instance, when caloric intake is restricted, the body may reduce thermogenesis to conserve energy, making it harder to lose weight. This is seen very often in diets that call for significant calorie restriction, and it creates an opposite effect as one would expect when they eat far fewer calories. Conversely, overfeeding can initially increase thermogenesis, but over time, the body adapts by becoming more efficient at storing excess energy as fat rather than burning it off as heat.

Nutrient partitioning, the process by which the body decides whether to store or burn incoming nutrients, is also influenced by weight gain. In individuals with obesity, the propensity to store nutrients as fat is heightened, partly due to hormonal changes. More glucose gets directed for fat storage and elevated levels of circulating fatty acids and altered adipokine profiles (hormones released by fat tissue) further promote fat storage over muscle building.

Stress influences eating behaviors and drives caloric intake. When an individual experiences stress, the body releases stress hormones like cortisol, which can increase appetite and cravings for high-calorie, palatable foods. This response is often termed "emotional eating," where food is used as a coping mechanism to manage negative emotions such as anxiety, sadness, or boredom. The consumption of comfort foods, typically rich in fats and sugar, can activate reward pathways in the brain, temporarily alleviating stress but leading to increased caloric intake and potential weight gain.

Semaglutide appears to have a significant effect on the neural circuits involved in reward and motivation, particularly in relation to food. It seems to dampen the pleasure response associated with eating, which can be a powerful tool for curbing overindulgence and unhealthy cravings. This effect is particularly useful for reducing cravings for poor food choices, although its impact on healthier options like fruits, vegetables, and whole grains may be less pronounced. While the precise mechanisms and consistency of these effects are still under investigation, imagine the possibilities if semaglutide helps you opt for broccoli over peanut butter! However, it's important to note that semaglutide's effect on the pleasure response to food is not permanent and a return of usual food preferences should be expected, unless, of course, you have begun to optimize your natural GLP-1 production.

Can semaglutide optimize hunger signals in an individual who is already metabolically healthy? For instance, imagine someone who does not wish to lose weight or alter their metabolic profile but would like to stop the habit of eating cookies after dinner every night. Is semaglutide a viable option in this scenario? Can diet and lifestyle changes geared toward GLP-1 optimization help?

In healthy individuals, GLP-1 levels are already tightly regulated to maintain energy balance and metabolic homeostasis. The effects of semaglutide on appetite in healthy individuals are less clear-cut. Some studies suggest that GLP-1 receptor agonists may also exert appetite-suppressing effects in healthy individuals, but the magnitude of these effects is generally less pronounced compared to those with metabolic disorders. Therefore, introducing a supraphysiologic dose of GLP-1 through medication may not have as dramatic an impact on appetite as it does in individuals with impaired GLP-1 function. However, even in healthy individuals, GLP-1 receptor agonists can still influence appetite and food intake. Studies have shown that these medications can increase feelings of fullness, reduce cravings, and decrease overall food intake, even in individuals without diabetes or obesity. This suggests that GLP-1 receptor agonists may have a broader therapeutic potential beyond their current indications. Meaning that semaglutide could potentially help reduce specific cravings, such as the desire for those cookies, by modulating the neural circuits involved in reward and motivation. The degree of appetite suppression in healthy individuals may vary depending on several factors, including the specific medication used, the dose, and individual differences in physiology and metabolism. Some individuals may experience a more pronounced reduction in appetite, while others may have a more subtle response.

Overall, the use of semaglutide for this purpose should be approached with caution. The effects are not permanent, and once the medication is discontinued, normal food preferences and cravings are likely to return. It's important to note that the long-term effects of GLP-1 receptor agonists on appetite and weight in healthy individuals are not yet fully understood. While these medications have been shown to be safe and effective in the short term, more research is needed to evaluate their long-term impact on appetite regulation and metabolic health. We will discuss some important questions regarding potential longer term effects in later chapters. This underscores the importance of lifestyle modifications geared toward GLP-1 optimization, which can help establish and maintain healthy habits.

CHAPTER 10: SUPERSTAR BLOOD GLUCOSE LEVELS

Semaglutide stands out as a groundbreaking treatment for type 2 diabetes due to its profound effects on blood sugar regulation. But here's the twist: even those without diabetes can benefit from better blood sugar management for overall health and metabolic wellness. This medication works by tackling two major issues: it boosts insulin secretion while suppressing glucagon, both of which support better blood glucose regulation. In this chapter, we'll dive into how semaglutide stimulates the pancreas to produce insulin when blood sugar levels rise and simultaneously inhibits glucagon release. Understanding these mechanisms will highlight semaglutide's pivotal role in managing hyperglycemia and preventing the complications associated with type 2 diabetes.

In type 2 diabetes, cells become resistant to insulin's signals, leading to an accumulation of glucose in the bloodstream. This chronic elevation of blood sugar, known as hyperglycemia, wreaks havoc on the body over time. Semaglutide helps break this vicious cycle, ensuring that insulin is released only when needed and preventing dangerous spikes in blood sugar. This comprehensive approach not only manages blood sugar levels but also offers significant protection against the long-term effects of diabetes.

Hyperglycemia causes extensive damage to various physiological systems and significantly increases the risk of life-threatening complications. One of the primary ways hyperglycemia inflicts harm is through its impact on blood vessels. Persistently high glucose levels can damage the endothelial cells lining the blood vessels, leading to atherosclerosis, or the hardening and narrowing of the arteries. This condition impedes blood flow and increases the risk of cardiovascular diseases, including heart attacks and strokes. The nervous system is another major target of hyperglycemia-induced damage. Elevated blood glucose can lead to diabetic neuropathy, a condition characterized by nerve damage that causes pain, tingling, and loss of sensation, particularly in the extremities. This nerve damage results from both direct glucose toxicity and impaired blood flow to the nerves. Over time, diabetic neuropathy can lead to severe complications, such as foot ulcers and infections, which in extreme cases may necessitate amputation.

Organ function can also be significantly impaired by prolonged hyperglycemia. The kidneys, for instance, are particularly vulnerable to high blood sugar levels, which can lead to diabetic nephropathy. This condition is characterized by damage to the glomeruli, the filtering units of the kidneys, resulting in proteinuria (the presence of protein in urine) and, ultimately, chronic kidney disease. If left untreated, diabetic nephropathy can progress to end-stage renal disease, necessitating dialysis or kidney transplantation.

The retina, the light-sensitive tissue at the back of the eye, is similarly susceptible to damage from hyperglycemia. Diabetic retinopathy occurs when high blood sugar levels damage the blood vessels in the retina, leading to vision problems and, in severe cases, blindness. This condition progresses through stages, starting with non-proliferative retinopathy, where small blood vessels leak fluid or hemorrhage, and advancing to proliferative retinopathy, where abnormal new blood vessels grow on the surface of the retina.

Beyond these specific complications, hyperglycemia contributes to a generalized state of inflammation and oxidative stress within the body. Chronic inflammation is a key factor in the development of various complications associated with diabetes, exacerbating cardiovascular diseases, neuropathy, nephropathy, and retinopathy. Oxidative stress, resulting from an imbalance between free radicals and antioxidants, further damages cells and tissues, compounding the detrimental effects of hyperglycemia.

While hyperglycemia is often associated with diabetes, the importance of glucose regulation extends far beyond those diagnosed with this condition. Everyone, regardless of their metabolic health status, requires effective blood sugar management to maintain overall health and well-being. Chronic high blood sugar levels can affect anyone, leading to subtle but significant damage over time. All the same damage, just on a more microscopic level. Unfortunately, this means that dysregulated glucose can go unknown for decades. With this, hand in hand comes increased risks of cardiovascular diseases, inflammation, oxidative stress, and impaired cognitive function. Ensuring stable blood sugar levels is crucial not only for preventing diabetes but also for supporting optimal energy levels, mental clarity, and long-term health. Proper glucose regulation helps avoid the rollercoaster of energy highs and lows, reduces cravings, and promotes a balanced metabolic state, making it a cornerstone of overall wellness.

Semaglutide's ability to lower and stabilize blood sugar levels can mitigate these risks, protecting the heart, nerves, and kidneys from the damaging effects of hyperglycemia. By improving glycemic control, semaglutide significantly enhances the quality of life for individuals with diabetes, reducing their risk of complications, boosting their energy levels, and allowing them to live fuller, healthier lives.

Beyond its intricate communication with the brain and gut, GLP-1 significantly influences the liver, a vital organ that serves as both a glucose storage facility and a distribution center, meticulously balancing the release and uptake of sugar to maintain energy homeostasis. Often under-appreciated, liver health plays a critical role in overall metabolic function and can account for a significant portion of metabolic derangements, as we discussed in the anatomy and physiology section. The liver stores excess glucose in the form of glycogen, a complex carbohydrate that acts as a reserve energy source. When blood sugar levels drop, the liver releases glycogen back into the bloodstream, ensuring a steady supply of fuel for the body's cells. This balancing act is orchestrated by a network of hormones, including GLP-1. Through its interaction with receptors on liver cells, GLP-1 helps maintain this equilibrium by suppressing the production of glucose. It achieves this by inhibiting gluconeogenesis, the process by which the liver creates glucose from non-carbohydrate sources.

Even for individuals who don't have diabetes, GLP-1 encourages a more measured release of insulin after meals, preventing the sharp spikes and subsequent crashes that often lead to fatigue, irritability, and cravings. This translates to steadier energy levels throughout the day, better focus, and potentially even reduced appetite due to more consistent satiety signals. This stabilization of blood sugar may be particularly beneficial for individuals with pre-diabetes, a condition where blood sugar levels are higher than normal but not yet high enough to be diagnosed as diabetes. By preventing these pre-diabetic levels from escalating, GLP-1 may help delay or even prevent the onset of full-blown type 2 diabetes, a significant health advantage.

It is also interesting to note that semaglutide's effects on blood sugar are not limited to fed states, but rather exert influence throughout the entire day, even in fasting states, contributing to overall glycemic control. Semaglutide effectively lowers fasting blood sugar levels by suppressing glucagon secretion from the pancreas, which in turn reduces the liver's glucose production overnight. This mechanism helps to prevent excessive morning hyperglycemia, a common challenge in diabetes management and non-diabetic metabolic derangement. Fasting glucose is increasingly being studied as a primary measure of longevity and overall metabolic health. Maintaining lower fasting glucose levels is associated with a reduced risk of metabolic syndrome, cardiovascular diseases, and other age-related conditions. By stabilizing blood sugar throughout the day, semaglutide not only aids in managing diabetes but also supports broader health and longevity goals. The continuous regulation of blood sugar facilitated by semaglutide underscores its potential to enhance metabolic health and improve long-term outcomes for individuals with and without diabetes.

As mentioned previously, after a meal, semaglutide stimulates a glucose-dependent insulin release. This means that the medication triggers insulin secretion only when blood sugar levels are elevated, preventing an excessive insulin spike and subsequent crash. Additionally, the delayed gastric emptying induced by GLP-1 agonism slows down the absorption of glucose into the bloodstream, contributing to a gentler rise in blood sugar levels after meals.

Whether you're fasting or eating, sitting or exercising, skipping carbs or indulging in French fries, GLP-1 improves the way your body processes glucose. Semaglutide harnesses these benefits to aid individuals in managing their blood sugar levels more effectively. For healthy individuals with normal blood sugar regulation and a healthy weight, the ideal level of GLP-1 receptor activity is naturally maintained by their bodies. This natural balance is key, restoring it being my primary motivation for writing this book.

The importance of striving for a natural, balanced GLP-1 response cannot be overstated. This is where the guidance provided in this book becomes invaluable. It arrives at a critical juncture in the national semaglutide journey, offering the necessary tools to build a healthy lifestyle that promotes optimal GLP-1 function. While semaglutide is a powerful tool for those needing immediate intervention, the long-term objective should be to support and enhance the body's natural metabolic processes. By focusing on diet, exercise, and overall wellness, you can achieve sustainable and lifelong weight loss and metabolic health. This approach not only maximizes the benefits of semaglutide but also maximizes your body's native responses and metabolic health, ensuring your ultimate expression of health and vitality.

CHAPTER 11: THE GLP-1 "SLOWDOWN" EFFECT

GLP-1 exerts a profound influence on the digestive process itself by slowing down the rate at which food leaves the stomach, a phenomenon known as delayed gastric emptying. Essentially, GLP-1 puts the brakes on your digestion, transforming it from a high-speed express train to a leisurely scenic route. This slowdown has several implications for weight loss and overall health.

First, delayed gastric emptying prolongs the feeling of fullness after a meal. When food lingers in the stomach longer, it triggers stretch receptors that signal to the brain that you're satiated. Stretch receptors, or mechanoreceptors, in the stomach play a critical role in signaling satiety and regulating food intake. These receptors are specialized nerve endings embedded in the muscular layers of the stomach wall that respond to mechanical changes, such as stretching or distention caused by food intake.

When food enters the stomach and begins to fill it, the stomach walls stretch, activating these mechanoreceptors. This activation sends afferent (sensory) signals via the vagus nerve to the nucleus tractus solitarius (NTS) in the brainstem. The NTS acts as a central processing hub, integrating these sensory signals and relaying them to higher brain centers, particularly the hypothalamus, a critical regulator of hunger and satiety, as we have learned. The mechanoreceptors in the stomach are sensitive to the degree of stretch, meaning that a greater volume of food will result in a stronger activation of these receptors. This increased activation translates to more robust and sustained signals being sent to the brain, indicating fullness and reducing the drive to continue eating. The continuous presence of food in the stomach, as seen with delayed gastric emptying induced by GLP-1, keeps these receptors activated for longer periods, thereby prolonging the sensation of satiety.

The prolonged presence of food in the stomach due to delayed gastric emptying enhances the activation of these stretch receptors, sending more persistent and robust signals of satiety to the hypothalamus. This continuous stimulation results in stronger and more sustained satiety signals, which can significantly alter eating behavior. The hypothalamus then integrates these signals with other inputs, such as hormonal signals from leptin and insulin, to modulate appetite and energy intake.

This signaling involves complex interactions between the gastrointestinal tract and the central nervous system, primarily through the vagus nerve. The vagus nerve, a crucial component of the parasympathetic nervous system, acts as a communication highway between the stomach and the brain. It is the longest cranial nerve, extending from the brainstem to various organs in the body, including the heart, lungs, and digestive tract. The vagus nerve plays a key role in the "rest and digest" functions of the parasympathetic nervous system, which counterbalances the "fight or flight" response of the sympathetic nervous system.

This heightened sense of fullness can help you feel satisfied with smaller portions, thus preventing overeating and promoting weight loss. The effects of delayed gastric emptying extend beyond simple volume-related stretch signals. By slowing gastric emptying, GLP-1 modulates the release of gut hormones such as

GLP-1 itself and peptide YY (PYY), which further enhance satiety. These hormones are secreted in response to the presence of nutrients in the intestines and act on the brain to reduce appetite and prolong the feeling of fullness.

When food is retained in the stomach for a longer period, GLP-1 ensures a more gradual and prolonged nutrient absorption process. This sustained presence of nutrients in the digestive tract leads to a more consistent and prolonged release of satiety hormones. PYY, another hormone released from the gut in response to food intake, acts on receptors in the brain to suppress appetite and prolong the sensation of fullness. Both of these hormones work synergistically to regulate hunger and food intake, making them powerful agents in appetite control.

By keeping food in the stomach longer, semaglutide facilitates a slower and more sustained release of these hormones. This multifaceted approach to enhancing satiety through delayed gastric emptying and hormonal modulation makes GLP-1 receptor agonists powerful tools in managing appetite and supporting weight loss. The result is a more controlled and manageable approach to eating, crucial for long-term weight management and metabolic health. Additionally, the slowed gastric emptying allows for a more effective nutrient absorption process in the intestines. This ensures that the body can extract and utilize vital nutrients from food more efficiently, which is particularly beneficial for individuals with nutrient absorption issues. The combination of enhanced satiety, stabilized blood sugar levels, and improved nutrient absorption creates a comprehensive strategy for achieving and maintaining a healthy weight and metabolic profile.

Second, delayed gastric emptying can stabilize blood sugar levels, even further elevating GLP-1's glucose stabilization efforts. When food is digested more slowly, glucose is released into the bloodstream at a more gradual pace, preventing the sharp spikes and subsequent crashes that often occur after consuming high-carbohydrate meals. Moreover, the gradual release of glucose means that insulin secretion from the pancreas is also more regulated. Instead of a rapid surge of insulin in response to a quick influx of glucose, the pancreas releases insulin more steadily. This gradual insulin release reduces the strain on pancreatic beta cells. Over time, this can help preserve the function of these cells, a likely critical factor in the development of diabetes.

Third, the GLP-1 digestive slowdown can significantly improve nutrient absorption. When food remains in the stomach and intestines for an extended period, the body has more time to extract valuable vitamins, minerals, and other essential nutrients. This extended interaction time between digestive enzymes and food allows for a more thorough breakdown of nutrients, enhancing their absorption into the bloodstream.

Digestive enzymes play a crucial role in the breakdown of macronutrients into their absorbable units: proteins into amino acids, fats into fatty acids and glycerol, and carbohydrates into simple sugars. The prolonged presence of food in the gastrointestinal tract ensures that these enzymes have ample opportunity to act on the food particles, increasing the efficiency of nutrient extraction. This process is particularly beneficial for individuals who struggle with malabsorption issues, such as those with certain gastrointestinal disorders or those who have undergone bariatric surgery. These conditions can significantly alter digestive efficiency and nutrient uptake, making the slower digestive process induced by GLP-1 receptor agonists like semaglutide especially advantageous.

Moreover, even individuals without overt malabsorption issues can benefit from improved nutrient absorption. Subclinical malabsorption, which may not present with obvious symptoms, is increasingly recognized as a common problem in modern diets. Factors such as the consumption of highly processed foods, low fiber intake, and the use of certain medications can impair nutrient absorption. Processed foods often lack the necessary enzymes and cofactors required for optimal digestion, and low fiber intake can reduce the transit time of food through the intestines, limiting the contact time for nutrient absorption. Certain medications, such as proton pump inhibitors and antibiotics, can also disrupt the balance of gut flora and enzyme activity, further impairing nutrient uptake.

By slowing gastric emptying, GLP-1 provides a potential therapeutic avenue to enhance nutrient uptake and improve overall nutritional status. The extended retention of food in the digestive tract allows for a more gradual and complete absorption of nutrients. Adequate intake of essential nutrients supports various metabolic processes, including energy production, cellular repair, and the synthesis of hormones and enzymes. For instance, sufficient absorption of vitamins and minerals such as iron, magnesium, and B vitamins is crucial for maintaining healthy metabolic function and preventing deficiencies that can lead to fatigue, impaired cognitive function, and other health issues.

The relationship between body weight and digestion speed is a complex and often misunderstood aspect of metabolic health. This topic has sparked considerable debate and intrigue within the scientific community, with some studies suggesting that individuals with obesity may have faster gastric emptying rates compared to their leaner counterparts. Such findings might initially seem counterintuitive, especially when considering the significant weight loss potential observed with semaglutide. However, the reality is that gastric emptying is a multifaceted process influenced by numerous factors, including the composition of the meal, hormonal signals, and individual physiological differences.

The composition of the meal is one of the most significant factors affecting this process. High-fat meals tend to slow gastric emptying due to the release of cholecystokinin (CCK), a hormone that stimulates the digestion of fats and proteins and signals the stomach to slow its emptying rate to allow more time for nutrient absorption. Conversely, liquid meals tend to empty more quickly than solid meals, as they require less mechanical breakdown and can pass through the pyloric sphincter more readily.

Individual differences in physiology also influence gastric emptying rates. Factors such as age, gender, physical activity level, and even psychological stress can impact the speed at which the stomach empties. For example, stress and anxiety can either accelerate or decelerate gastric emptying depending on the individual's response to stress. Regardless of the precise relationship between obesity and gastric emptying, it is evident that semaglutide can significantly slow down gastric emptying in individuals regardless of their body weight. By extending the time food remains in the stomach, semaglutide enhances the activation of stretch receptors and the prolonged release of satiety hormones. This not only helps individuals feel fuller for longer periods but also leads to more stable blood glucose levels by modulating the rate at which glucose enters the bloodstream.

Overall, studies are inconclusive regarding the transit rates of obese individuals. Some have reported significant differences, while others have reported no significant difference in gastric emptying rates between obese and non-obese individuals, or even slower emptying rates in those with obesity. These discrepancies may be due to variations in study designs, methodologies, and the populations studied. Factors such as the type of meal consumed (solid vs. liquid), the macronutrient composition of the meal, and the specific metrics used to measure gastric emptying can all influence outcomes and contribute to the variability in findings.

One plausible explanation for these varied results is the alteration in gut hormones observed in individuals with obesity. Obese patients often exhibit impaired feedback mechanisms between the stomach and the brain. These hormonal imbalances can disrupt the normal regulation of hunger and satiety, potentially leading to altered gastric emptying rates. Additionally, changes in the structure and function of the stomach muscles, such as decreased motility or increased compliance, may further affect the rate at which food leaves the stomach. Lastly, gut health must be considered.

Obesity has been associated with alterations in gut microbiota, which play a crucial role in nutrient absorption. The gut microbiota can influence the digestion and absorption of various nutrients, including fats and carbohydrates, by modulating the production of digestive enzymes and affecting the integrity of the gut barrier. These alterations may lead to changes in the way the body absorbs certain nutrients, contributing to the metabolic dysregulation seen in obesity.

Overall, this slower, more mindful approach to digestion offers a wealth of potential benefits[2]. It allows for more efficient nutrient absorption, ensuring that your body receives the full spectrum of vitamins, minerals, and other essential compounds from your food. It promotes a stable blood sugar level, reducing the risk of insulin resistance and metabolic dysfunction. It even fosters a healthier gut microbiome, the bustling community of microbes that play a crucial role in digestion, immunity, and overall well-being. This is a long-term investment in metabolic health. By optimizing digestion and nutrient absorption, it lays the foundation for a healthier, more resilient body. It's a shift towards a more sustainable way of eating, one that nourishes both body and mind.

When we adopt a GLP-1 lifestyle, we align more closely with the body's natural processes and homeostasis, which can mitigate potential side effects and maximize the benefits of this hunger hormone. By focusing on enhancing endogenous GLP-1 production through methods we will discuss later, we can achieve similar benefits with far fewer drawbacks. Understanding the balance between therapeutic benefits and potential side effects is crucial in the management of metabolic disorders. Optimizing native GLP-1 levels offers a more sustainable and tolerable approach, reducing the risk of severe gastrointestinal symptoms while still providing significant improvements in metabolic health. We've explored semaglutide's multifaceted benefits, its profound effects on appetite suppression, glucose regulation, and the GLP-1-induced slowdown of digestion. Each of these mechanisms

---

[2] Side note: It isn't all positive. For some individuals, this alteration in digestive pace can lead to nausea, sometimes progressing to vomiting, bloating and distention. Constipation can be another result. These side effects must be weighed on an individual risk vs. benefit scale.

plays a critical role in managing weight and improving metabolic health.

As we move forward, it's essential to address the potential downsides of semaglutide therapy. While the benefits of GLP-1 receptor agonists are significant, they are not without their challenges. The next chapters will focus on side effects, ranging from mild gastrointestinal issues to more severe concerns. Understanding these effects is crucial for managing and mitigating, ensuring that patients can achieve the maximum benefits of semaglutide with minimal discomfort.

Additionally, we will explore more serious side effects, including the potential impact on the pancreas, thyroid, and other organs. We'll examine the evidence surrounding these risks, providing a balanced view of the benefits and drawbacks of semaglutide therapy. By comprehensively addressing both the advantages and the potential pitfalls of semaglutide, I aim to equip you with the knowledge needed to make informed decisions about your health. This holistic approach will help you navigate the complexities of metabolic health and harness the full potential of GLP-1 in a safe and effective manner.

SECTION III: SIDE EFFECTS & DOSING

CHAPTER 12: MY PERSONAL BURNING QUESTIONS

Moving forward wouldn't be complete without the crucial step of delving into the side effects associated with semaglutide, going above and beyond the common discomforts of nausea and constipation. I want to start this section with the questions that I sought to answer, the concerns I have for these drugs as a physician and lifelong pursuer of health.

Understand that not all of these are negative. Side effects are just that, on the side of the primary purpose of the medication. They are not necessarily harmful nor beneficial. These are simply questions that I raised to my own research. We will explore concerns about rebound weight gain and the potential impacts on metabolic function. We will discuss the potentially permanent effects you may expect from optimizing your GLP-1 levels. This knowledge will equip you to navigate the complexities of your weight loss journey, maximizing the benefits while mitigating the risks, all within safe and reasonable parameters.

Firstly, what can we expect from long-term changes in appetite with semaglutide? Does newfound satiety continue with a permanent shift, does appetite come back stronger than before, or is there a darker undercurrent to satiety in the first place? For many, it appears the latter. While the initial days of appetite suppression may seem bright, beautiful and full of hope for a new beginning in one's relationship with food, it appears that a shadow often lingers. Many individuals continue to experience alarming decreases in appetite. This sounds potentially positive however maintaining a significantly reduced appetite post-weight loss can be detrimental. The body needs to adjust and increase calorie intake to stabilize at the new, lower weight. Persistent low appetite can hinder this stabilization, leading to a metabolic state where the body perceives ongoing caloric deficit, eventually triggering mechanisms that promote weight regain. This phenomenon, often termed "rebound weight gain," is one of the most dreaded side effects of semaglutide therapy. This is all secondary to the "post fat loss injury" event that the body has undergone. Losing fat mass is a traumatic event and, though maybe surprising to you, the body is looking for signals of safety in the environment at this stage. Continuing with zero appetite, caloric restriction and potential nutrient deficiencies with mild malnutrition is not the safety signal the body needs following a fat loss event. Much more on this fat loss injury to come in a later chapter.

A phenomenon known as "rebound hunger" can occur, where individuals experience a surge in appetite once they stop taking semaglutide. The once-muted cravings resurface with a vengeance, creating a chorus of desire for the very foods that semaglutide had tamed. This heightened sense of hunger can lead to overconsumption and a rapid regain of the lost weight, undoing the progress made during the medication period. The portions that once seemed satisfying may now appear insufficient, leaving individuals with a persistent feeling of deprivation and a strong urge to eat more.

The reasons behind the rebound effect observed with semaglutide cessation are multifaceted, involving intricate threads of physiology, psychology, and environmental factors. As we discussed previously, chronic exposure to supraphysiologic levels of GLP-1 likely leads to a downregulation of GLP-1 receptors in the brain. The brain's adaptation to high levels of GLP-1 during treatment can result in a diminished response once the medication is discontinued. The brain's receptors, having been continuously stimulated by the medication, become less sensitive to the hormone. This reduced sensitivity can lead to increased hunger and a stronger desire for food, as the brain's usual signals of fullness and satiety are blunted. This is a likely case as these type of feedback loops exist in most other hormone and endocrine cycles.

The fluctuations in appetite underscore the complexity of semaglutide's effects on the body's hunger and satiety mechanisms. The variability in response among different individuals highlights that the effects on appetite and weight regulation are not uniformly predictable. Factors such as individual physiology, baseline metabolic state, and the body's adaptive mechanisms, like thermogenic changes, all contribute to this variability. The interplay between GLP-1 and other hunger hormones complicates the picture. Remember, the rapid weight loss induced by semaglutide can trigger compensatory mechanisms in the body designed to protect against starvation. These mechanisms include a decrease in metabolism and an increase in appetite stimulation via ghrelin. Ghrelin increases in response to calorie restriction and weight loss, driving hunger and food intake. The elevated levels of ghrelin post semaglutide can make it significantly harder to maintain weight loss, as the body aggressively signals the need for increased energy intake. We know that semaglutide's modulation of GLP-1 temporarily alters the balance and that the body's natural regulatory mechanisms will eventually reassert themselves, it is in this reassertion where individual response varies.

For many, semaglutide provided a period of respite from their challenging food behaviors, allowing them to experience a sense of control over their appetite and eating habits. However, the return of these underlying issues can be disheartening and overwhelming. The psychological burden of dealing with re-emerging emotional eating patterns can lead to increased stress and anxiety, further complicating efforts to maintain a healthy GLP-1 lifestyle.

The sense of reliance on semaglutide for appetite control can also affect self-efficacy, or the belief in one's ability to manage their own health and eating behaviors. When the medication is discontinued, individuals may feel less confident in their ability to maintain the healthy habits they developed while on the drug. This decrease in self-efficacy can contribute to a cycle of negative emotions and behaviors, making it even more challenging to sustain weight loss and healthy eating patterns.

In modern society, where high-calorie foods are easily accessible and heavily marketed, the once-dulled cravings may reignite with greater intensity. The allure of "forbidden" foods, which might have been manageable while motivated and excited on semaglutide, can become almost irresistible. This can lead to episodes of overeating or binge eating, undoing the progress made during treatment and potentially leading to weight regain.

Second, what might one expect from changes in food preference long term? As it turns out, one of the most intriguing effects of semaglutide is its ability to subtly alter food preferences, particularly in those with a penchant for less healthy options. This shift isn't about a sudden distaste for your favorite foods, but rather a decrease in the intensity of cravings, especially for sugary snacks, carbs and greasy fast food! The science behind this change lies in the way semaglutide affects the brain's reward system, which we previously discussed. By modulating dopamine signaling, the medication can dampen the pleasure response associated with these high-calorie foods. Dopamine is a neurotransmitter that plays a critical role in the brain's reward and pleasure centers. Foods that are high in sugar and fat typically cause a significant release of dopamine, which reinforces the desire to consume these foods again and again. Semaglutide appears to alter this dopamine response, reducing the reinforcement, making these foods less compelling. This doesn't mean you'll suddenly hate chocolate or find pizza repulsive, but the pull of these foods may become less intense, making it easier to choose a healthier option. For instance, the desire for a full-on cheeseburger might diminish, allowing you to be more content with a burger salad. This shift in food preference is not just a temporary effect but has the potential for long-term change, especially if supported by consistent GLP-1 lifestyle modification.

The alteration in food preferences induced by semaglutide is also linked to changes in the gut-brain axis. The gut-brain axis is a bidirectional communication system between the gastrointestinal tract and the central nervous system. GLP-1 is a key player in this axis. By slowing gastric emptying and modulating nutrient absorption, semaglutide changes the gut's feedback to the brain. This feedback involves hormones and neural signals that inform the brain about the types and quantities of nutrients being processed, which can influence food choices and eating behaviors.

Moreover, research has established quite convincingly that the gut microbiota can impact food preferences. It's simple enough, really. Healthy lifestyle choices like eating colorful vegetables and ferments as well as exercising and getting outside all support the proliferation of good guy gut bacteria. All the same, Burger King and couch surfing support the growth of bad guy gut bacteria. Once established, these bacteria just want more of what helped them grow in the first place, and they actually send signals through the gut-brain axis to tell you what you want to eat. Semaglutide's effects on the gut microbiota could potentially contribute to the shift towards healthier food choices by promoting a gut environment that favors beneficial bacteria. In this way, semaglutide may indirectly support better food preferences and overall metabolic health.

Another aspect to consider is the psychological impact of weight loss and improved health on food choices. As individuals shed pounds and experience enhanced physical and mental well-being, they often naturally gravitate towards healthier foods. The positive reinforcement of feeling better and achieving weight loss goals can strengthen a preference for nutritious, lower-calorie foods over time. Utilizing tools like this to shift your mindset is a powerful method toward a healthier lifestyle.

As an example, I frequently encourage my clients to adopt fasting regimens due to their multifaceted health benefits for metabolic health, digestion, fat loss, eating pattern adherence, and mental fortitude. One secondary benefit of fasting, which I refer to as "positive action multiplication," is particularly noteworthy. Typically, after fasting, individuals feel a sense of accomplishment (and hunger). What is amazing is that they often feel their body deserves quality nourishment after working hard to fast, thus they wish to choose a high-nutrient meal. They don't want to "waste" their fast by breaking it with unhealthy food! This is a prime example of positive psychology at work, reinforcing healthy eating habits through the natural rewards of their efforts.

Third, I had wondered about permanent or long-lasting changes in digestion or nutrient absorption in the gut with semaglutide. Does the GLP-1 slowdown have a positive long term effect? As we know, this deliberate slowdown profoundly impacts the gut's intricate workings. On one hand, as we know, it can be a boon for nutrient absorption. However, this slower pace can also have its drawbacks, culminating in those side effects previously briefly discussed (gas, bloating, diarrhea and constipation).

Additionally, the long-term impact on the gut microbiome is still an area of ongoing research. We know for sure that GLP-1's effects on the microbiota are positive, while the jury is still out on the supraphysiologic dosing seen with semaglutide. The truly vast importance of this community of bacteria is just beginning to reveal itself to mainstream medicine; it is remarkable the power that our microbiome has over every health process. Given the complexity and importance of the microbiome, any medication that alters its composition warrants careful consideration.

Fourth, does semaglutide have an effect on fat storage or adipose tissue behavior? It appears semaglutide is able to reach deep into the body's energy reserves and into the very landscape of fat storage, causing a potentially powerful shift and a rebalancing of the scales (pun intended).

Imagine fat as a vast reservoir of military resources in war time. There are seemingly plenty of resources, yet, assuring that nothing goes to waste seems prudent. This is essentially how the body treats fat and is how so many of us end up with far too many "resources" for our own personal wars. Semaglutide has some independent action here that is definitely worth mentioning. The medication acts like a shrewd strategist on the opposing side, deploying a multi-pronged attack to deplete these reserves. By curbing appetite and reducing food intake, semaglutide limits the raw materials needed for fat production, like cutting off supply lines. Semaglutide also infiltrates communication lines, disrupting the intricate processes that govern the storage of more fat.

One of these pathways is lipogenesis, the process through which excess carbohydrates are converted into triglycerides, the building blocks of fat. Under the influence of semaglutide, the activity of enzymes involved in lipogenesis decreases, effectively slowing down the fat-building factory. This means that less dietary carbohydrate is transformed into stored fat, reducing the overall accumulation of adipose tissue. Simultaneously, semaglutide rallies the body's own defenses, boosting lipolysis, the breakdown of stored fat for energy. This process is critical for mobilizing fat reserves and utilizing them to meet the body's energy demands. By enhancing lipolysis, semaglutide increases the rate at which fat is metabolized, opening the floodgates of the reservoir and releasing pent-up energy to fuel the body's activities. This dual action—reducing fat storage and increasing fat burning—creates a powerful one-two punch that can lead to significant and sustained fat loss.

Beyond these direct effects on fat metabolism, semaglutide also influences adipose tissue behavior. Adipose tissue is not just a passive storage site for energy. In fact, it actually functions more like an active endocrine organ, secreting various hormones and inflammatory mediators. In individuals with obesity, adipose tissue often becomes dysfunctional, contributing to chronic inflammation and insulin resistance. Semaglutide's ability to reduce adiposity can help mitigate these adverse effects, improving overall metabolic health. Moreover, as we have learned, semaglutide's impact on insulin sensitivity facilitates better utilization of glucose, further diminishing the need for fat storage.

Studies have shown that semaglutide can preferentially target visceral fat, the deep abdominal fat that wraps around organs and is associated with a higher risk of metabolic disease. Unlike subcutaneous fat which lies just under the skin, visceral fat poses a significant threat due to its proximity to vital organs. This type of fat is highly metabolically active and releases inflammatory markers and free fatty acids directly into the liver through the portal vein. This process exacerbates insulin resistance, contributes to fatty liver disease, and increases the risk of cardiovascular diseases. By reducing visceral fat, semaglutide helps lower these risks, promoting better overall health. Visceral fat is a true scourge of modern society and a significant contributor to our epidemic of fatty liver and metabolic disease.

The mechanism by which semaglutide targets visceral fat involves several pathways. Firstly, its appetite-suppressing effects reduce overall caloric intake, creating an energy deficit that forces the body to utilize stored fat for energy, of which the body targets visceral fat for priority removal. Secondly, like previously mentioned, semaglutide enhances lipolysis, the breakdown of fat stored in adipocytes, particularly in visceral fat cells. Moreover, semaglutide reduces the secretion of adipokines from visceral fat. Adipokines are signaling proteins released by fat tissue that can have pro-inflammatory effects, contributing to metabolic disorders and chronic inflammatory disease. By decreasing visceral fat, semaglutide reduces the production of these harmful proteins, thereby lowering inflammation and improving insulin sensitivity as well as overall health. The reduction in visceral fat not only improves metabolic parameters but also has significant implications for cardiovascular health. Visceral fat is closely linked to increased cardiovascular risk, as it contributes to atherosclerosis, hypertension, and dyslipidemia. By targeting and reducing visceral fat, semaglutide helps mitigate these risks, supporting cardiovascular health and reducing the likelihood of heart disease.

As fat stores dwindle, waistlines shrink, organs become free from highly inflammatory visceral fat and the risk of metabolic complications diminishes, semaglutide delivers a victory not just on the scale, but also within the intricate landscape of our cells and tissues. Talk about a multifaceted attack on fat!

Fifth, what can we expect to see from metabolic shifts in the long term? Semaglutide adjusts the tempo and intensity of various metabolic processes and we know that GLP-1 leads to a harmonious balance of energy utilization and storage. Does semaglutide do the same?

One of semaglutide's key impacts on metabolism lies in its ability to enhance insulin sensitivity. I have repeated this fact multiple times, I hope you are starting to see the inevitable entanglement between insulin sensitivity and health. Insulin, as a reminder, is the hormone responsible for ushering glucose from the bloodstream into cells, playing a pivotal role in energy metabolism. In individuals with insulin resistance, cells become less responsive to insulin's signals, leading to elevated blood sugar levels and impaired energy utilization. This increased sensitivity not only improves blood sugar control but also has a ripple effect on other metabolic pathways.

As mentioned, studies have shown that semaglutide can increase resting energy expenditure, the amount of energy the body uses at rest to maintain basic functions like breathing and circulation. This means that individuals on semaglutide may burn more calories throughout the day, even when they're not actively exercising. The mechanisms behind this increase in energy expenditure are not fully understood, but they may involve changes in mitochondrial function, the cellular powerhouses responsible for energy production. If this turns out to be true, it has massive implications for GLP-1's role in health and longevity. Mitochondria are incredibly important to our health, mood, and disease status. They are responsible for generating the energy needed for cellular functions, and any enhancement in their efficiency can significantly boost metabolic health. Modern sources state approximately 90% of current disease states are mitochondrial in origin. Quite literally anything you can do to increase the health, efficiency, power or numbers of your mitochondrial colony will go a long way to promoting overall health-span. For the purposes of this book, I cannot give mitochondrial health the time it deserves. I would suggest reading a book specifically written about this subject if your interest is piqued.

Moving on, semaglutide may influence protein turnover, the balance between protein synthesis and degradation. Maintaining a healthy protein turnover rate is essential for muscle maintenance. Muscle mass, like fat, actually functions in an organ like fashion as well by improving overall metabolic function, fat burning potential and energy utilization.

The comprehensive metabolic effects of semaglutide suggest that it orchestrates a broad, beneficial impact on the body's energy balance. By enhancing insulin sensitivity, increasing energy expenditure, and possibly improving mitochondrial and muscular function, semaglutide promotes a more efficient and healthier metabolic state. This multifaceted approach not only supports weight loss but also contributes to overall metabolic health, potentially reducing the risk of metabolic disorders and improving quality of life.

These reflections aimed to provide a comprehensive understanding of the long-term implications of semaglutide, emphasizing the need for thoughtful discontinuation strategies and sustained lifestyle modifications for lasting health benefits, while also understanding that this drug really does hold some magic promises.

CHAPTER 13: COMMON SIDE EFFECTS

It is important that anyone considering treatment with semaglutide understand the nature of the most common side effects. Although serious side effects are frightening and you should understand them, common side effects are just that. They happen to many individuals, in fact, most people will experience some version of one or more of these. For the most part these are minor discomforts, annoyances and small drawbacks. However, it remains important for you to prepare yourself as to avoid any potential heartache (or bellyache, in this case) or early cessation of treatment prior to desired results.

In the landscape of GLP-1 agonist therapy, gastrointestinal side effects are a common topic of discussion among both patients and healthcare providers. The risk of some version of gastrointestinal upset is quite high and should be presented as a reality vs. a distant side effect. Fortunately (or unfortunately, depending on individual fate) the spectrum of these common disorders varies widely, with some people experiencing minor, irritating effects such as transient mild morning nausea or mild diarrhea following meals.

Diarrhea and constipation frequently emerge as notable concerns to the users of semaglutide. This occurs when the balance of fluid absorption and secretion in the intestines is disrupted. As you know, GLP-1 agonists slow gastric emptying, increasing the amount of time food spends in the stomach before entering the intestines. This delayed transit will affect digestive processes and fluid balance, interestingly, individuals lean on opposite sides of the fence on this issue. Some appear to produce more fluids in response, resulting in diarrhea. Others appear to absorb more fluids from the large intestine, resulting in constipation. Currently, we are operating blindly in our ability to parse out which patients might have which adverse gastrointestinal event.

Clinical trials and observational studies demonstrate that generally speaking, diarrhea is a very common side effect and not one of particular concern. In most cases, it is described as mild to moderate in severity and tends to diminish as the body adjusts to the medication. For instance, studies have shown that gastrointestinal side effects are most pronounced during the first few weeks of treatment. These symptoms typically decrease in frequency and severity over time as patients acclimate to the drug. Similar patterns have been observed with other GLP-1 agonists, such as liraglutide and exenatide. The transient nature of diarrhea suggests that it is often a manageable side effect rather than a persistent or severe issue. The body at first reacts to the initial up-regulation of GLP-1 by increasing and overshooting the typical physiologic response. However, in its perpetual effort to achieve and maintain homeostasis, the body finds a way to balance the fluid alterations occurring by semaglutide's actions.

Now of course, diarrhea can be distressing and may impact adherence to GLP-1 agonist therapy. Educating yourself about this potential can help set realistic expectations and improve adherence. Understanding that these symptoms are usually temporary and manageable can alleviate anxiety and encourage continued use of the medication. There are a few management strategies that can be quite helpful to minimize discomfort and ensure effective and continued use of semaglutide. Starting with a lower dose and gradually increasing it can help mitigate gastrointestinal side effects. This approach allows the body to adjust to the medication more gradually, reducing incidence and severity. I encourage you to begin a GLP-1 lifestyle right away, as this will immediately help regulate bowel movements and quell side effects. In the initial stages, avoiding foods that are known to irritate the gastrointestinal tract, such as spicy foods, can also be beneficial.

Given that the nature of the diarrhea is not infectious, there is likely no issue with taking over-the-counter anti-diarrheal medications, such as loperamide, to provide symptomatic relief for persistent concerns. However, these should be used under the guidance of a healthcare provider to ensure they do not interfere with the therapeutic effects of GLP-1 agonists.

There are a few situations which warrant special consideration. While GLP-1 induced diarrhea is paired with pre-existing gastrointestinal conditions, such as irritable bowel syndrome (IBS) or inflammatory bowel disease (IBD), diarrhea can be more severe and persistent. In such cases, the discomfort and impact on quality of life may necessitate a reevaluation of the treatment regimen. Additionally, severe or prolonged diarrhea can lead to dehydration, electrolyte imbalances, and nutritional deficiencies. Those experiencing these complications should seek medical attention promptly to manage these risks and optimize the strategy to continue with effective utilization of semaglutide.

Most can continue the medication with appropriate strategies to mitigate diarrhea. Implementing effective management techniques can help with navigating this aspect of GLP-1 agonist therapy, ensuring optimal therapeutic outcomes and improved metabolic health.

Constipation is also a common gastrointestinal side effect of semaglutide, which can be a significant concern for many. There are a few reasons for this. As mentioned previously, the delay in gastric emptying induced by semaglutide is one of its most effective mechanisms for controlling blood glucose levels and appetite. However, when food moves more slowly through the large intestine, it can lead to increased water absorption from fecal matter, resulting in harder stools and more difficult bowel movements.

Similar to diarrhea, one often experiences constipation shortly after initiating semaglutide therapy, as the body adapts to the medication's effects and recalibrates toward homeostasis. This can lead to discomfort, bloating, and abdominal pain. The severity of constipation varies among individuals, with some experiencing mild symptoms while others face more significant challenges that can affect their quality of life. In clinical trials, constipation was reported by a substantial number of participants, highlighting its prevalence as a side effect.

GLP-1 receptors act on the vagus nerve and in the enteric nervous system, enhancing the release of acetylcholine, a neurotransmitter that modulates peristalsis, the wave-like muscle contractions that move food through the digestive tract. This is how semaglutide effectively prolongs the digestive process, which can hinder the efficient passage of waste. Interestingly, this works in a similar fashion to opiate medications, which also significantly slow down peristalsis. These medications are quite notorious in the medical world for causing concerning levels of constipation.

Moreover, semaglutide's influence on gut hormones further complicates the picture. The hormone peptide YY (PYY), which is co-released with GLP-1, also slows gastric emptying and intestinal motility. Elevated levels of PYY contribute to the sensation of satiety but can exacerbate constipation. Additionally, semaglutide likely alters the gut microbiota, these changes have untold effects on gastric motility.

Management of semaglutide-induced constipation typically involves dietary and lifestyle modifications. Increasing dietary fiber intake, staying well-hydrated and considering a stool softener are first-line strategies to alleviate symptoms. It is also important to keep communication lines open with your healthcare provider regarding bowel habits. I specifically mention this because patients are often too embarrassed to discuss this openly and frequently. However, it's important to do so.

Nausea and abdominal pain are among the most commonly reported side effects of semaglutide, understanding the underlying mechanisms can provide insight into these often uncomfortable symptoms. Nausea occurs in a significant proportion of patients starting semaglutide therapy, with some studies reporting an incidence as high as 44%. The nausea primarily stems from the delayed gastric emptying. By slowing down the rate at which food leaves the stomach, semaglutide extends the period that food remains in the stomach, which can lead to a sensation of fullness and, consequently, nausea.

Abdominal pain associated with semaglutide use is reported in up to 20% of patients. This pain can range from mild to severe and may present as cramping, bloating, or generalized discomfort. The pain is often linked to the same mechanisms that cause nausea—delayed gastric emptying and changes in gastrointestinal motility. Additionally, semaglutide's effects on the gastrointestinal tract can lead to the accumulation of gas and changes in bowel habits, which can further contribute to abdominal pain.

In a similar approach to other side effects, gradual dose escalation is a key approach, allowing the body to adjust slowly to the medication. Starting with a lower dose and incrementally increasing it helps to minimize the severity of nausea and abdominal pain. This gradual titration helps the body reach that homeostasis we have discussed previously, which lessens the drug's negative effects on the gastrointestinal system. It is also advisable to eat smaller, more frequent meals rather than large meals, which can help manage the symptoms by reducing the burden on the stomach.

For most individuals, the gamut of gastrointestinal side effects of semaglutide tend to diminish over time as their bodies adjust to the medication. However, if these symptoms persist or become severe, it is essential to consult with your healthcare provider. In some cases, adjusting the dose or switching to a different medication may be necessary to improve tolerability. Understanding the underlying mechanisms and employing appropriate management strategies can help mitigate these symptoms or at the very least, aid with your understanding and realistic expectations of the experience. By gradually increasing the dosage and adopting dietary modifications, most can continue to benefit from semaglutide's therapeutic effects while minimizing discomfort.

Hypoglycemia, or low blood sugar, is a potential side effect of semaglutide, particularly when used in combination with other glucose-lowering medications, as would be the case with diabetics. This of course should come as no surprise, given that glycemic control is a primary effect of semaglutide's efficacy for diabetes and obesity. Despite its glucose-dependent action, the risk of hypoglycemia still exists, however, it is not a normal response to the drug. It appears the vast majority of hypoglycemic episodes with semaglutide are iatrogenic, or caused by an exogenous medication that likely should have been tailored to account for semaglutide's presence. Externally injected insulin or sulfonylureas, for instance, will cause hypoglycemia independent of blood glucose levels. When used in conjunction with semaglutide, the additive effect can lead to excessive lowering of blood glucose.

Hypoglycemia is characterized by a range of symptoms that result from the body's attempt to raise blood glucose levels. Early signs include shakiness, sweating, rapid heartbeat, anxiety, hunger, and irritability. If blood sugar levels continue to fall, symptoms can progress to confusion, drowsiness, and even loss of consciousness. Severe hypoglycemia is a medical emergency and requires immediate treatment to prevent serious complications. The physiologic mechanisms behind hypoglycemia involve the interplay of various hormones and metabolic pathways. When blood glucose levels drop, the pancreas reduces insulin secretion and increases glucagon release. Glucagon stimulates the liver to convert stored glycogen into glucose, releasing it into the bloodstream to raise blood sugar levels. Additionally, the adrenal glands release adrenaline, which also promotes glucose production by the liver. These counter-regulatory mechanisms are essential for preventing severe hypoglycemia.

However, in individuals with diabetes, these counter-regulatory responses are often impaired, especially after prolonged use of insulin or other medications that affect glucose metabolism. For example, repeated episodes of hypoglycemia can blunt the body's response to low blood sugar, making it more difficult to recognize and treat subsequent episodes. This condition, known as hypoglycemia unawareness, increases the risk of severe hypoglycemia and its associated complications.

If you are concurrently using glucose lowering medications, the recommendation from your healthcare provider will more than likely be to reduce the dose of said medication. Of course, as always, careful patient selection and frequent examinations and monitoring at home are of critical importance. Most diabetics are aware of the signs and symptoms of hypoglycemia and how to manage it, however, education when on semaglutide is also critical. Quick-acting sources of glucose, such as glucose tablets and fruit juice should be readily available for treating mild to moderate hypoglycemia. For severe hypoglycemia, a glucagon injection or intravenous glucose in a medical facility may be necessary.

Tachycardia, or a heart rate over 100 beats per minute, is another potential side effect of semaglutide, warranting careful consideration. This cardiovascular effect is significant due to the potential implications for overall cardiovascular health.

Amazingly, GLP-1 receptors even exist within the heart and blood vessels, otherwise known as the cardiovascular system. The exact mechanism by which semaglutide induces tachycardia is not fully understood, but several hypotheses exist. One possibility is simply that GLP-1 directly influences heart rate, seems obvious, however, no-one knows why that might be the case. If so, this effect would be mediated through the autonomic nervous system, particularly by increasing sympathetic nervous system activity, which accelerates the heart rate. This would be a fascinating finding because, as we know, GLP-1 has direct effects on the parasympathetic nervous system, particularly through the vagus nerve. Interestingly, the vagus nerve controls lowering of the heart rate, so this opposing autonomic nervous system effect based on particular tissues would be a fascinating revelation. However, it is possible that GLP-1 can activate both sides of the autonomic nervous system, including the heart rate lowering effects of the parasympathetic nervous system in cardiac tissue. In fact, this notion is supported, as there are studies showing that GLP-1 receptor agonists can influence heart rate variability, which is a measure of parasympathetic activity in the heart.

In clinical trials, the increase in heart rate associated with semaglutide use was generally modest, but it was consistent across different studies and patient populations. For example, in the *SUSTAIN* clinical trials, an increase in heart rate of about 2-4 beats per minute was observed in patients treated with semaglutide compared to those receiving placebo. This is a modest increase, but any increase in heart rate can create extra work for the heart, as well as extra oxygen utilization. This increase in heart rate would go unnoticed by the vast majority, but those with symptomatic cardiac disease would be wise to discuss semaglutide with their healthcare provider.

Headaches are a common side effect reported by individuals taking semaglutide, and understanding the underlying mechanisms and impacts can provide insight into this often bothersome symptom. The exact pathophysiology of semaglutide-induced headaches is not entirely understood, but several potential mechanisms have been proposed. One possibility involves the central nervous system. GLP-1 receptors are expressed in various regions of the brain, including those involved in pain perception and modulation. Activation of these receptors can influence neurotransmitter release and neuronal excitability, potentially leading to headaches.

Another contributing factor may be changes in blood glucose levels. Fluctuations in blood glucose levels, especially if they occur rapidly, can trigger headaches. This is particularly relevant in the initial stages of treatment when the body is adjusting to the new medication regimen.

Vascular changes induced by semaglutide might also contribute to headaches. The GLP-1 receptors in blood vessels can cause vasodilation, or opening of the blood vessels. While this can be beneficial for cardiovascular health by reducing blood pressure, it can also lead to headaches in some individuals due to changes in cerebral blood flow.

Management here is fairly simple; stay well-hydrated, consider any over-the-counter pain relievers you are comfortable taking for headache, monitor blood sugar levels and blood pressure regularly, see your healthcare provider if its serious enough and consider adjusting the dose of semaglutide. As is the case with most side effects on this medication, starting with a lower dose and gradually increasing allows the body to acclimate to the medication.

Fatigue is a commonly reported side effect of semaglutide, and its underlying mechanisms are multifaceted, involving both physiologic and psychologic components. One of the primary ways semaglutide may cause fatigue is through significant changes in blood glucose levels, particularly in the initial stages of treatment. Blood glucose fluctuations are known to cause fatigue, and this would be especially true if your one of the unlucky few who experiences hypoglycemia on semaglutide, as low blood sugar levels are well-known to cause feelings of weakness and tiredness.

The effect of semaglutide on gastric emptying also plays a role in the sensation of fatigue. Every time you eat on semaglutide, the meal is treated like a miniature Thanksgiving dinner. Gastric motility is slowed, therefore, more time is spent digesting, more energy is diverted to this process and the more exhausted you feel.

Furthermore, the central nervous system effects of semaglutide may contribute to fatigue. GLP-1 receptors in the brain influence neurotransmitter release and neuronal activity, which could potentially lead to fatigue. The brain's response to changes in blood glucose levels and hormone fluctuations can also affect overall energy levels and alertness.

Psychological factors must also be considered. The process of adjusting to a new medication and managing its side effects can be mentally exhausting. The stress and anxiety associated with starting a new treatment regimen, particularly one as impactful as semaglutide, can lead to feelings of fatigue. Additionally, the lifestyle changes you will be needing to undergo alongside semaglutide can initially contribute to tiredness as the body adapts.

We've explored the less serious yet still impactful side effects of semaglutide, focusing on their mechanisms and management strategies. We discussed gastrointestinal issues like constipation, nausea, and abdominal pain, emphasizing how these symptoms are related to the medication's effects on gastric emptying and digestion. Additionally, we examined common side effects such as headaches, fatigue, and the potential for tachycardia, detailing the physiologic pathways involved. This chapter aimed to provide a balanced view of managing these side effects to ensure comfort and adherence to semaglutide therapy.

CHAPTER 14: SERIOUS SIDE EFFECTS

Though serious side effects are by their very nature uncommon, they warrant careful consideration for anyone considering semaglutide. It is critical to undertake a thorough medical history with your healthcare provider, as the commonality within these side effects is that they occur far more amongst those with preexisting disease.

Pancreatitis stands out as an alarming potential side effect. Pancreatitis is an inflammation of the pancreas, a crucial organ involved in both digestive and endocrine functions. The pancreas produces digestive enzymes that help break down food in the intestine and hormones like insulin and glucagon that regulate blood sugar levels. Inflammation of the pancreas can disrupt these functions and cause digestive issues, while also leading to severe abdominal pain and potentially life-threatening complications like ischemia and death of the tissue.

The exact mechanism by which GLP-1 agonists might increase the risk of pancreatitis remains under investigation. One proposed mechanism involves the overstimulation of pancreatic beta cells, leading to increased enzyme production and potential cellular stress. Another hypothesis suggests that GLP-1 agonists might cause changes in the exocrine function of the pancreas, increasing the risk of enzyme leakage and subsequent inflammation. Additionally, GLP-1 agonists might induce changes in the gut microbiota, which could influence pancreatic health indirectly. Of these, the second appears most likely as altered pancreatic function and enzyme over production and leakage is a commonly seen etiology of pancreatitis in the world of medicine. It stands to reason, additionally, that over stimulation of GLP-1 could lead to this complication as well.

Clinical trials and observational studies have reported instances of pancreatitis in patients taking GLP-1 agonists, though the overall incidence appears to be relatively low. For instance, a review of clinical trial data for liraglutide noted an increased incidence of pancreatitis compared to placebo. However, subsequent large-scale observational studies and meta-analyses have provided mixed results, with some indicating a slight increase in risk and others finding no significant association. Case reports have highlighted instances where patients developed acute pancreatitis shortly after initiating GLP-1 agonist therapy. Symptoms typically include sudden, severe abdominal pain, nausea, vomiting, and elevated levels of pancreatic enzymes such as amylase and lipase. Imaging studies, such as abdominal ultrasound or CT scans, often confirm the diagnosis by showing inflammation and swelling of the pancreas. It is important to note that case reports hold very little weight of scientific rigor as compared to large randomly controlled trials and best yet, meta-analyses. Given that the meta-analyses are more optimistic and inconclusive is a positive sign.

One must consider who is most susceptible to pancreatitis in the first place. It is highly likely that individuals who suffer pancreatitis after GLP-1 agonist therapy were already at an extremely elevated risk of pancreatitis as compared to a control individual with normal metabolic health. Given the epidemic proportions of metabolic dysfunction we are seeing in modern society and the role of the pancreas in metabolic health, this appears to be a reasonable and safe conclusion. It is also noteworthy that metabolic disease is a vast spectrum, very likely with many years, even decades, of subclinical non-optimal health occurring before any frank disease rears its ugly head. Semaglutide could simply be the straw that broke the proverbial camel's back. Certain other factors may predispose individuals to an increased risk of pancreatitis when using GLP-1 agonists, including a history of pancreatitis, presence of gallstones, excessive alcohol consumption and high triglyceride levels. Of course, all of these are associated with poor metabolic health.

No-one with great metabolic health should be prescribed a GLP-1 agonist in the first place, so we really do not have a choice but to ford these intrepid waters. For those prescribed GLP-1 agonists, close monitoring is essential. Patients should be educated about the signs and symptoms of pancreatitis and instructed to seek immediate medical attention if they experience severe abdominal pain. Pancreatitis becomes a big problem quickly, it is not one to fuss about with or to deal with once you're home from vacation!

If pancreatitis is suspected, clearly stopping semaglutide is paramount. From there, pancreatitis is mostly a palliative disease, meaning that modern medicine really has nothing to offer you but supportive treatment. A pancreatitis patient will be fasting to rest the pancreas, given intravenous fluids to remain hydrated, offered pain management and any potential underlying etiology will be addressed, such as in gallstone pancreatitis or with critical triglyceride levels. Most cases of drug-induced pancreatitis resolve with appropriate medical management, but severe cases may require more intensive interventions, such as endoscopic procedures or surgery.

The potential risk of pancreatitis must be weighed against the substantial benefits of GLP-1 agonists in managing diabetes and obesity. For many patients, the metabolic improvements offered by these medications outweigh the relatively low risk of pancreatitis. However, individualized risk assessment and vigilant monitoring are crucial to ensuring patient safety. While the association between GLP-1 agonists and pancreatitis remains a complex and somewhat contentious issue, understanding the potential risks and implementing careful monitoring strategies can help mitigate adverse outcomes. By staying informed and proactive, healthcare providers can harness the benefits of GLP-1 agonists while minimizing the risks, which at this time appears a prudent strategy.

The pancreas and gallbladder communicate with one another and each help to coordinate the dance of proper digestion. Each has their role in proper metabolic health, therefore, it only stands to reason that GLP-1 agonists present a risk to the state of the gallbladder. First, some etymology. Anything gallbladder related is denoted "chole", so gallbladder stones and inflammation are known as cholelithiasis and cholecystitis, respectively. The procedure to undergo removal of the gallbladder is know as a cholecystectomy. Understanding the link between GLP-1 agonists and conditions like cholelithiasis, cholecystitis, and the subsequent risk of requiring cholecystectomy is essential for optimizing patient outcomes and minimizing adverse effects.

Cholelithiasis is a condition that can be influenced by various factors, most notably for our purposes, including after rapid weight loss. Gallstones are hardened deposits that can form in the gallbladder, and their presence can lead to significant health issues. Rapid weight loss is known to increase the risk of gallstone formation because it can lead to increased cholesterol levels in bile, which can precipitate into stones. Since GLP-1 agonists promote significant weight loss, patients using these medications may be at an elevated risk for developing cholelithiasis. Studies have shown that patients on successful semaglutide therapies have a higher incidence of gallstones compared to the general population. This simply goes with the territory of quickly losing weight. Again, like pancreatitis, are we seeing cholelithiasis in patients who were already a setup to develop stones in the first place? My suspicion, same as before, is absolutely yes.

Cholecystitis is the inflammation of the gallbladder, often resulting from a gallstone blocking the cystic duct. When gallstones obstruct the flow of bile, it can lead to inflammation and infection of the gallbladder. This risk is particularly relevant for patients on GLP-1 agonists, given the higher likelihood of rapid weight loss and subsequent gallstone formation. Observational studies and clinical trials have reported cases of cholecystitis in patients undergoing this treatment, necessitating careful monitoring and prompt intervention when symptoms arise. This condition can cause severe abdominal pain, fever, and digestive disturbances. Cholecystitis is a ticket to a cholecystectomy, more often than not. There does not appear to be any evidence suggesting that GLP-1 agonists actually increase the risk of cholecystitis, outside of cholelithiasis, but simply that increasing the formation of stones increases the risk of an inflammatory condition within the gallbladder.

Cholecystectomy, the surgical removal of the gallbladder, becomes necessary when cholelithiasis and cholecystitis cause significant symptoms or complications. The relationship between GLP-1 agonists and the increased need for cholecystectomy is a critical consideration for healthcare providers. Cholecystectomy is often performed for any symptomatic gallstone disease, and very often for any bout of cholecystitis. This is due to the fact that symptomatic gallstone disease is likely to occur at a future point, so current medical belief is a bit of a "no time like the present" approach to removing the gallbladder. Clinical data indicate that a notable proportion of patients on GLP-1 agonists have undergone cholecystectomy due to gallstone-related complications. Again, it is very likely in my opinion that these patients either already had gallstones or were already pre-determined to develop gallstones, and semaglutide simply ushered the process along.

Having a cholecystectomy is not simply a matter of taking care of the inevitable, it is a significant event in that one is losing an important organ of digestion and metabolism. The gallbladder stores bile produced by the liver, a critical player in the metabolism of fats. The liver is not meant to efficiently produce bile to be released at the right moments for digestive harmony, therefore, individuals who are post cholecystectomy have a serious issue digesting fats and often have to avoid this important macronutrient in their diets. This is not the topic of this book so I won't dive any deeper than this, just suffice to say that although this is an extraordinarily common procedure, it is my professional opinion, in an ideal world it would not be. The gallbladder is far from a vestigial organ; it is metabolic disease that often leads to its excision from the body which in turn creates a vicious cycle of down spiraling metabolic health.

The most effective management strategy to reduce the risks associated with GLP-1 agonist therapy concerning gallbladder health is a gradual, sustained weight loss rather than rapid weight reduction, which significantly helps to minimize the risk of gallstone formation. Of course, utilizing optimal natural GLP-1 response vs. semaglutide therapy goes a long way in controlling the rapidity of fat loss and potential gallstone formation within the gallbladder. When using semaglutide, a balanced approach ensures that patients can continue to benefit from these medications while avoiding these more serious downsides.

An increased risks of ocular disease, particularly retinopathy, is a significant and potentially disastrous side effect that has been demonstrated in individuals on semaglutide. Retinopathy is a disease affecting the retina of the eye. The retina contains the vast majority of the blood flow to the eyes, as well as many vital components of vision, such as the rods and cones. Diabetic retinopathy is a progressive eye disease caused by damage to the blood vessels in the retina due to prolonged high blood glucose levels. It is a leading cause of blindness in adults and manifests through stages, ranging from mild non-proliferative retinopathy to proliferative retinopathy, where abnormal blood vessels grow on the retina's surface. These changes can lead to vision loss and eventual blindness if not managed effectively.

The relationship between GLP-1 agonists and retinopathy is complex. Clinical trials have indicated both potential benefits and risks associated with these medications. On one hand, improved glycemic control with GLP-1 agonists can reduce the overall risk of diabetic complications, including retinopathy. On the other hand, there have been concerns that rapid improvements in blood glucose levels may transiently worsen retinopathy. Though the issue is certainly complex, there is likely a correlating phenomenon at play which we have already experienced earlier in this chapter. It is quite likely that a worsening retinopathy is only seen in individuals who already have advanced disease within the retina. Similar to our findings with worsened cholelithiasis and pancreatitis, what can be viewed as “GLP-1 agonists cause retinopathy” is actually, “GLP-1 agonists hasten existing significant disease”.

This has already been elucidated to some degree. Some studies have suggested that patients with pre-existing severe diabetic retinopathy may experience a progression of the condition when starting GLP-1 agonist therapy. This phenomenon is thought to be related to the rapid lowering of blood glucose levels, which, although beneficial in the long term, might temporarily destabilize retinal blood vessels. Such changes underscore the importance of gradual glycemic improvements and close monitoring of ocular health in patients with significant retinopathy.

Clinical trials such as the *SUSTAIN-6* study have provided valuable insights into the potential ocular risks associated with GLP-1 agonists. In this trial, an increased incidence of diabetic retinopathy complications was observed in patients treated with semaglutide compared to those receiving a placebo. This finding prompted further investigation and highlighted the need for careful patient selection and monitoring.

It is important to note that the observed increase in retinopathy risk was primarily associated with patients who had a history of severe retinopathy at baseline and experienced substantial and rapid reductions in HbA1c. This suggests that the risk is not inherent to the GLP-1 agonists themselves but rather related to the dynamics of glycemic control.

Like with any other potential complication, it is important to scale the physiologic effects of semaglutide, to gradually ramp up treatment, to have frequent ocular examinations and to collaborate and participate fully with all members of your medical team while on or considering semaglutide therapy.

One of the most hot button topics surrounding semaglutide has been the concern over malignancies of the thyroid gland. Thyroid cancer is a serious concern that has been linked to the use of GLP-1 agonists in some studies, particularly a potential to increase the risk of medullary thyroid carcinoma (MTC), a rare but aggressive form of thyroid cancer. This concern stems from preclinical studies in rodents, which have shown an increased incidence of MTC in animals treated with GLP-1 agonists. These findings led to a black box warning by the FDA for certain GLP-1 agonists, cautioning against their use in patients with a personal or family history of MTC or multiple endocrine neoplasia syndrome type 2 (MEN 2). Again, in patients with a significant preexisting concern.

The exact mechanism by which GLP-1 agonists might contribute to thyroid cancer development is not fully understood. One hypothesis suggests that these drugs may stimulate the growth of C-cells in the thyroid gland, which are responsible for producing the hormone calcitonin. Increased calcitonin levels have been observed in some patients treated with GLP-1 agonists, raising concerns about potential C-cell hyperplasia and the development of MTC. However, the relevance of these findings in humans remains a subject of ongoing research and debate.

Epidemiological studies in humans have provided mixed results. Some studies have not found a significant increase in thyroid cancer risk among patients using GLP-1 agonists, while others suggest a potential association. For instance, a review of post-marketing surveillance data did not show a clear increase in thyroid cancer cases among users of these medications compared to the general population. However, given the rarity of MTC, detecting a small increase in risk requires long-term, large-scale studies. Unfortunately, it is difficult to feasibly attain large studies or meta-analyses in such a rare disease.

Regular monitoring of thyroid function and calcitonin levels may be warranted in patients treated with GLP-1 agonists, especially those at higher risk. This gives healthcare providers a clue that thyroidal c-cells are proliferating abnormally, a hallmark of any malignancy. Although routine calcitonin screening is not universally recommended due to its limited predictive value and the rarity of MTC, it can be considered in certain high-risk individuals.

While the potential risk of thyroid cancer is a serious consideration, it must be weighed against the substantial benefits of GLP-1 agonists in managing diabetes and promoting weight loss. For many patients, the advantages of improved glycemic control, reduced cardiovascular risk, and significant weight loss outweigh the relatively low risk of developing thyroid cancer.

Recent clinical trials, including the *SUSTAIN-6* and *PIONEER 6* trials, have demonstrated that semaglutide can provide significant benefits for kidney health, especially in individuals with type 2 diabetes. These studies found that semaglutide significantly reduced the risk of new or worsening nephropathy (kidney disease). Specifically, semaglutide reduced the risk of persistent macroalbuminuria by 36% and showed a 21% reduction in the risk of new or worsening nephropathy in another trial.

Semaglutide's kidney benefits are believed to be multifactorial. Firstly, its ability to lower blood sugar levels reduces the strain on the kidneys. Elevated blood glucose can damage the delicate structures within the kidneys over time, leading to diabetic nephropathy. By maintaining better glycemic control, semaglutide helps protect the kidneys from this damage. Secondly, semaglutide's effect on weight loss can also indirectly benefit kidney health. Obesity is a significant risk factor for kidney disease, and weight loss can reduce this risk and improve overall kidney function.

However, not all findings on semaglutide and kidney health are positive. This is a chapter on serious side effects, after all. There have been post-marketing reports of acute kidney injury (AKI) in patients taking semaglutide. Not surprisingly, the vast majority of these findings have been associated with individuals with pre-existing chronic kidney disease (CKD). Most of what we are seeing with negative effects on the kidneys is secondary to loss of fluids and electrolytes, for example from diarrhea. These effects are minor and inconsequential for healthy kidneys, however, they can cause damage in organs with pre-existing disease.

There is ongoing research to determine if GLP-1 receptor agonists have a direct impact on renal tissues. The expression of GLP-1 receptors in the kidneys suggests potential direct effects that might contribute to nephrotoxicity under certain conditions. These reports continue to highlight the importance of close monitoring, particularly in individuals with existing kidney disease. Symptoms such as a decrease in urine output, swelling in the legs or ankles, and unexplained fatigue should prompt immediate medical attention as they may indicate worsening kidney function. Although AKI is a significant clinical concern, these reports are rare and almost exclusively a concern for those with CKD. The decision to use semaglutide in patients with CKD should be made with careful consideration and close monitoring of kidney function tests, including serum creatinine and glomerular filtration rate (GFR). Like with everything else we've discussed, selection of appropriate individuals is key.

Clearly, individualized risk assessment and patient-centered care are essential in making informed decisions about GLP-1 agonist therapy. For patients with low baseline risks, the benefits of these medications can be substantial. In contrast, for those with higher risk, alternative treatment options may be necessary. Patient selection and careful monitoring become absolutely paramount for all minor and major side effects we have discussed thus far. For some, this means not being a candidate for GLP-1 agonist therapy, though I do believe this individual is fairly rare. A prudent approach to reduce any complication is to aim for gradual improvement in blood glucose levels and gradual weight loss. Plus, always remember, an optimized GLP-1 lifestyle comes with practically zero risk, even for individuals with pre-existing diseases.

CHAPTER 15: DOSING TO EFFECT

Imagine two climbers preparing to embark on a challenging ascent up a steep mountain. Tomorrow, they will begin their race to the top, with a significant monetary award for the victor. They have completed all preparations: months of training, sleeping well on their travels, setting up base camp, checking the weather forecast and acclimating to their new environment. They've spent thousands on top gear from REI and Patagonia. Feeling fully educated and physically prepared, they are ready to take on the summit.

The next morning, at the trailhead, the two climbers exchange well wishes and begin their journey. One sets off with a dead sprint, eager to reach the top quickly. The second climber, however, takes a moment to assess his body, mind, and spirit. He sets a pace that is challenging yet sustainable, one he can maintain indefinitely. Who wins in this scenario?

Ok, maybe that was a little too obvious and a "tortoise and the hare" rip-off, but it illustrates an important point about embarking on a medication like semaglutide. The reality is that any approach toward weight loss must be a journey if there is an expectation for sustainability. There are countless stories of people in a rush to lose weight that took them three decades to accumulate. Some lose weight, most don't. Of those who do, the vast majority put it back on. Even worse, with every subsequent fat loss event, the body becomes more resistant to having another event occur successfully. This is part of the fat loss injury that we will discuss in a later chapter.

One is rarely successful by sprinting towards the summit. The more sensible approach is well calculated steps that allow the body to adjust to the altitude and terrain. A wise starting dose for semaglutide is 0.25mg. This is a tentative first step, an introduction to the medication's potent effects. This careful approach is like spending a few days at base camp, doing some light hiking. It is designed to acclimate the body to the medication, reducing the risk of side effects and optimizing its therapeutic benefits. As the body adapts, the dosage is gradually increased over several weeks, like our climber steadily ascending towards higher altitudes. This incremental approach serves several critical purposes and allows titration of the medication to occur, which limits side effects.

The gradual dose escalation allows healthcare providers to fine-tune the treatment plan based on individual response and tolerability. Each person's journey with semaglutide is unique, and the optimal dose will vary. By gradually increasing the dose, the sweet spot can be identified, where the medication is most effective while side effects remain minimized. The idea is to find the lowest possible dose that maximizes an individual patient's beneficial effects.

This gradual titration not only reduces the potential for side effects but also allows the body's various systems to adjust to semaglutide's metabolic effects. The body needs time to adjust to the metabolic changes that occur as semaglutide mimics the incretin hormones that the body naturally produces. Furthermore, the phased increase in dosage helps optimize the therapeutic effects of semaglutide, enhancing its ability to suppress appetite and promote weight loss. As the dose increases, semaglutide's impact on hunger signals becomes more pronounced. This stepwise approach is crucial for balancing efficacy and tolerability, ensuring that patients can reap the maximum benefits of the medication without overwhelming their system.

Several studies have demonstrated that gradual dose escalation can significantly reduce the incidence and severity of gastrointestinal side effects. For instance, a study published in The Lancet examined the safety and efficacy of semaglutide in a population of patients with type 2 diabetes. The study found that starting with a dose of 0.25 mg and gradually increasing it to 1 mg or higher over several weeks helped to mitigate nausea and vomiting, leading to better overall tolerance of the medication.

Similarly, another clinical trial reported in the *Journal of Clinical Endocrinology & Metabolism* confirmed that patients who underwent a gradual dose escalation experienced fewer gastrointestinal side effects compared to those who started at a higher dose. The study highlighted that a slower titration schedule allowed patients to adapt more comfortably to the medication, resulting in improved adherence and better glycemic control. These findings have been elucidated in real-world clinical practice as well.

When semaglutide is introduced at a low dose, it gently begins to influence insulin secretion from the pancreas. This low starting dose helps the body to start processing glucose more efficiently without overwhelming the insulin-producing beta cells. Over time, as the dosage is increased incrementally, the pancreas gradually increases its insulin output in response to meals. This gradual adjustment helps the body to avoid sudden drops in blood sugar levels, which can occur if insulin production is ramped up too quickly. Additionally, the process of managing glucagon secretion needs to be finely balanced to prevent hypoglycemia. The gradual increase in semaglutide dosage gives the liver time to adjust its glucose output, maintaining stable blood sugar levels without causing dangerous lows.

Moreover, semaglutide affects on the brain's regulation of appetite and satiety needs to be introduced gradually to allow the brain's neurocircuitry to adjust, preventing potential issues such as severe hunger suppression or an imbalance in other hormonal signals related to food intake. This gradual increase in dosage allows adjustment to the changing levels of appetite suppression. Starting with a low dose, the body begins to experience subtle changes in hunger and satiety. Patients may notice a slight reduction in their usual hunger patterns, making it easier to adhere to healthier eating habits. Over time, as the dosage is incrementally raised, the effects become more pronounced. Additionally, the gut-brain axis is allowed to adjust without overwhelming the system, leading to more consistent and stable therapeutic outcomes.

The cardiovascular system, including the heart and blood vessels, also needs time to adjust to these changes. Gradual titration ensures that these systems adapt smoothly, minimizing the risk of adverse cardiovascular events like hypotension or tachycardia.

Maybe most importantly, this stepwise approach supports sustainable weight loss. Rapid weight loss can often be followed by rebound weight gain if the body is not given time to adjust nor heal from the injury of fat loss. The gradual increase in semaglutide dosage helps to ensure that weight loss is steady and sustained. Patients are more likely to develop and maintain healthy eating behaviors as they adjust to the new appetite cues provided by the medication. This gradual process helps to cement lifestyle changes that are critical for sustainable weight management.

The practical benefits of this strategy are significant. Patients who experience fewer side effects are more likely to continue with their treatment regimen, which is crucial for achieving long-term glycemic control and weight loss. Moreover, improved adherence translates to better clinical outcomes, including reduced HbA1c levels and sustained weight reduction.

In essence, the semaglutide cycle is a journey of discovery, a gradual ascent towards a healthier weight and a revitalized life. It's a process that requires patience, perseverance, and a willingness to listen to your body's signals as well as your healthcare provider's advice. By working closely with them and following the recommended dosing schedule, you can harness the full potential of the medication and achieve your weight loss goals in a safe and sustainable way. Remember, patience is a virtue!

CHAPTER 16: "MEGA" DOSING

Although starting small and escalating the dose is critical, semaglutide is meant to provide a level of GLP-1 agonism that surpasses anything naturally produced. This is a deliberate strategy designed to maximize therapeutic benefits. By exceeding the body's natural production of GLP-1, these medications can more effectively activate GLP-1 receptors throughout the body, amplifying the hormone's effects.

In healthy individuals, GLP-1 levels fluctuate throughout the day, peaking after meals and returning to baseline levels between meals. These fluctuations are tightly regulated to maintain energy balance and metabolic homeostasis. However, in individuals with type 2 diabetes or obesity, GLP-1 levels may be impaired, leading to dysregulated appetite, elevated blood sugar levels, and other metabolic disturbances. Administering supraphysiologic doses of semaglutide effectively compensates for this deficiency, restoring and even enhancing the beneficial effects of GLP-1. The higher levels of GLP-1 achieved with these medications can more effectively initiate the beneficial effects of the medication.

With semaglutide, unlike native GLP-1, there is a steady and elevated level of activity. This overrides the body's natural fluctuations and can have profound effects on various aspects of metabolism. For instance, the increased insulin secretion helps to lower blood sugar levels more effectively, while the suppression of glucagon release reduces the amount of glucose produced by the liver. The slowing of gastric emptying helps to moderate the rate at which glucose enters the bloodstream, preventing postprandial spikes in blood sugar levels. The impact on appetite is particularly significant. By enhancing the feeling of fullness and reducing hunger, supraphysiologic doses of GLP-1 agonists help patients to eat less and make healthier food choices. This is crucial for individuals struggling with obesity, as it addresses overeating driven by dysregulated hunger signals. The reduction in cravings for high-calorie foods further supports weight loss and helps in the adoption of a more balanced diet.

Moreover, cardiovascular improvements are amplified with semaglutide, allowing the body to essentially "catch up" on years of poor cardiovascular health. As mentioned previously, these medications have been shown to improve cardiovascular outcomes, an essential consideration given the increased risk of heart disease in patients with type 2 diabetes and obesity.

Studies have shown that the peak GLP-1 levels achieved with Ozempic (with a larger dose, 1 mg) are approximately 5-10 times higher than those seen after a meal in healthy individuals. For Wegovy (2.4 mg), the peak levels are even more pronounced, estimated to be around 15-20 times higher than physiologic levels. These supraphysiologic levels are thought to be necessary to achieve the significant weight loss and glycemic control observed in clinical trials. As discussed previously, it is likely that overweight individuals do not have the same GLP-1 levels nor the same response as their leaner counterparts. It is highly plausible that a thin individual's GLP-1 response is inherently stronger, potentially 5-20 times greater than that of an overweight individual. Therefore, by introducing semaglutide, we may simply be making the playing field a little more even, enhancing GLP-1 levels to match those naturally found in healthier individuals.

The supraphysiologic dosing of semaglutide has been shown to be safe and effective in the short term, leading to substantial weight loss and improved glycemic control. However, the long-term effects of chronic exposure to elevated GLP-1 levels are still being studied. One area of concern is the impact on pancreatic beta-cell function. While semaglutide stimulates insulin secretion, there is a theoretical risk that chronic stimulation could lead to beta-cell exhaustion or dysfunction over time. Another concern is the risk of developing pancreatitis or other gastrointestinal complications on a more long term basis. Lastly, rebound weight gain is issue number one on everyone's mind, and there is still question to what effects a supraphysiologic dose has on incidence of rebound weight gain in semaglutide users. Although clinical trials have shown that semaglutide is generally well-tolerated, with a relatively low incidence of severe side effects, the long-term safety profile is still being established.

Despite these potential concerns, the supraphysiologic dosing of semaglutide in Ozempic and Wegovy represents a novel approach to harnessing the therapeutic potential of GLP-1. By exceeding the body's natural production of this hormone, these medications can effectively address the underlying biologic mechanisms that contribute to obesity and type 2 diabetes. The significant weight loss and glycemic control observed in clinical trials offer new hope for individuals struggling with these chronic conditions, providing a powerful tool in the fight against metabolic disease.

CHAPTER 17: "MICRO" DOSING

Microdosing is all about taking tiny doses of a drug—doses much lower than what's typically used for treatment. The idea is to tap into some of a drug's benefits while sidestepping the full blown physiologic and many of the possible side effects that often come with standard doses. Initially, microdosing gained fame in psychiatry with substances like LSD and psilocybin, where it was reported to boost cognitive function and emotional well-being without a psychedelic trip. Now, this intriguing approach is making waves in the world of metabolic health, GLP-1 receptor agonists included. Imagine enjoying the perks of these powerful medications without the common side effects. That's the promise of microdosing!

Exploring the benefits of microdosing in the psychiatric world, lets take Sarah, a high-achieving professional in her mid-thirties, who found herself struggling with anxiety and creative blocks that were taking a toll on her work and personal life. Despite trying various conventional treatments, she couldn't shake the feeling of being stuck in a mental fog. One day, she stumbled upon an article about the emerging practice of microdosing psilocybin—the active compound in magic mushrooms. Intrigued by the potential to enhance cognitive function and emotional well-being without experiencing any psychedelic trip, Sarah decided to explore this uncharted territory.

She started with just a fractional dose of what would be considered a recreational amount, once every few days. The dose typically used for microdosing psilocybin does not provoke any conscious awareness to the patient. The idea is that it is working in the background, on a subconscious level. To her surprise, within weeks, she noticed subtle yet profound changes. Her anxiety levels began to drop, replaced by a calm clarity that she hadn't felt in years. Creative ideas flowed more freely, and her productivity soared. The microdoses didn't alter her consciousness, but they gently lifted the fog, allowing her to see and think more clearly.

Sarah's experience is not unique. As more people experiment with microdosing psilocybin, anecdotal reports of enhanced focus, emotional resilience, and overall well-being have surfaced. Scientists have taken notice, and preliminary studies now back up these anecdotal claims. Research indicates that microdosing could help with mood regulation, cognitive flexibility, and even neurogenesis—the growth of new neurons in the brain.

Sarah's journey with microdosing psilocybin opened up a new chapter in her life, filled with possibility and renewed vigor. It also illustrated a broader shift in how we approach treatment—favoring gentle, incremental changes over aggressive interventions. This emerging strategy of microdosing holds incredible promise, offering a pathway to improved health and well-being that harmonizes with the body's natural rhythms.

This has captured the attention of researchers, clinicians and practitioners within other fields. In metabolic health, we are seeing a significant uptick in interest in microdosing GLP-1 receptor agonists. Just as with psilocybin, the goal is to harness the therapeutic benefits in a background role.

Similarly, in cardiology, microdoses of beta-blockers have been used to manage certain types of arrhythmias. These low doses can effectively control heart rhythm abnormalities without causing the profound bradycardia (excessively slow heart rate) that often accompanies higher doses. This approach allows for effective treatment while minimizing the potential for negative side effects, thereby improving patient compliance and outcomes.

In the context of metabolic health, microdosing represents a significant shift in treatment paradigms. By offering the benefits of drugs like semaglutide while minimizing their often challenging side effects, microdosing could make these treatments more accessible and tolerable for a broader range of patients. This includes those with mild metabolic disorders, those particularly sensitive to medications or those simply looking for background assistance in their weight loss efforts. These lower doses can provide therapeutic effects needed to improve metabolic health while reducing the incidence of adverse reactions.

Embracing microdosing in metabolic health could lead to more personalized and patient-friendly treatment plans. It opens the door to utilizing powerful medications like semaglutide in populations that may have previously been unable to tolerate standard doses, or those without the necessary pathology to warrant typical dosing strategies. This approach not only enhances patient comfort and adherence but also broadens the potential for these medications to positively impact public health. By carefully calibrating microdoses to individual needs, healthcare providers can optimize the balance between efficacy and tolerability, ultimately leading to better health outcomes and improved quality of life for patients.

Preclinical studies have provided valuable insights into the potential benefits of microdosing GLP-1 agonists. Animal models have shown that fractional doses can improve glycemic control and reduce body weight. These studies suggest that partial activation of GLP-1 receptors can produce significant metabolic benefits while minimizing adverse effects. Research indicates that fractional doses can achieve meaningful improvements in HbA1c and body weight. Although the degree of improvement may be less pronounced than with standard doses, the trade-off in reduced side effects and increased tolerability can make microdosing a preferable option for many patients. Case studies and patient testimonials also highlight the practical benefits of this approach, with individuals reporting better adherence to treatment and improved overall health outcomes. These findings suggest that microdosing could play a significant role in the future of metabolic health management. Anecdotal evidence from patients and healthcare providers further highlights the potential benefits of microdosing. Some patients have reported improved adherence to treatment and better overall quality of life.

One of the key mechanisms by which microdosing GLP-1 agonists may exert their effects is through partial receptor activation. By administering fractional doses, it is possible to achieve a level of receptor activation that provides therapeutic benefits without fully saturating the receptors. This partial activation can enhance insulin sensitivity, improve glucose uptake, and modulate appetite without triggering the full spectrum of effects associated with higher doses. Microdosing also allows for gradual physiologic adaptation. This slow acclimatization can help mitigate the initial shock to the system that can occur with standard dosing, even the low doses typically started with. This is particularly important for drugs that affect multiple physiological systems, such as GLP-1 receptor agonists.

Given the potent effects of these drugs, there is a strong rationale for exploring microdosing as a viable therapeutic approach.

Microdosing can potentially harness metabolic benefits while minimizing side effects that can detract from the overall patient experience. The key to successful microdosing lies in finding the optimal balance between efficacy and tolerability. It may be possible to achieve a more subtle modulation of brain signals, reducing hunger and promoting satiety without completely suppressing appetite.

Currently, there is no established or widely accepted microdosing protocol for semaglutide in medical practice. However, some healthcare providers and compounding pharmacies are experimenting with significantly lower doses based on their clinical judgment and patient need. A typical approach might begin with doses as low as 0.05 mg once a week. The key is to start with a very low dose to assess individual tolerance and minimize the risk of side effects. Over time, the dose can be increased every 2-4 weeks based on how well the patient tolerates the medication and the observed effectiveness. For instance, each adjustment might involve increasing the dose by 0.05 mg.

Let's look at a sample dosing schedule. I offer this sneak peak because the dosing strategy is actually the same, whether standard or microdosing. Let's specifically look at a microdosing setup where a patient could start with 0.05 mg once a week for the first four weeks. We would then continue monitoring, journaling and counseling regarding the positive and negative effects occurring at this dose. With a discussion between patient and provider, the decision could be made to step up the dose, at this point increasing to 0.1 mg once a week for the next four weeks. After the same counseling and consideration for adjustment, the dose could be increased to 0.15mg once a week for another four weeks. The decision could be made from here to increase the dose weekly or continue straight into the more standard starting dose of 0.25 mg. The titration process is a nuanced art form. Ongoing monitoring and dose adjustment are crucial components and patients should be regularly evaluated for changes in glycemic control, weight, and overall health. Adjustments to the dosing regimen may be necessary based on these assessments to ensure optimal therapeutic outcomes. Regular consultation with a provider is essential throughout this process!

While the concept of microdosing GLP-1 agonists is still emerging, there is a growing body of preclinical and clinical evidence supporting its potential benefits. Early studies suggest that even at lower doses, GLP-1 agonists can improve glycemic control and promote weight loss, albeit to a lesser extent than standard therapeutic doses. However, the reduction in side effects and improved patient tolerability could make microdosing a preferable option for certain patient populations. On the back of highly positive clinical and anecdotal evidence, I fully expect the future of microdosing to be extremely bright. Particularly in the case of a medication like semaglutide, where administration is not urgent. In fact, for semaglutide and many other medications, the "low and slow" approach has serious benefits and little downsides. As the microdosing concept takes hold, I believe we will see it emerge as a primary means of initiating administration of any non-urgent medications and I strongly urge you to consider it if you are on the fence regarding a full dose of semaglutide.

CHAPTER 18: STOPPING THE MEDICATION, FOREVER

The semaglutide journey is much like navigating a well-charted course, with distinct phases that include a beginning, middle, and crucially, an end. While the promise of sustained weight loss and improved metabolic health can make the idea of indefinite use appealing, it's important to recognize that semaglutide, like any medication, is not meant for lifelong use. Successfully discontinuing the medication and transitioning to a natural GLP-1 lifestyle involves a thoughtful, well-structured plan, emphasizing gradual changes and sustainable health practices.

The decision of when to discontinue semaglutide is a deeply personal and oft confusing one. It will absolutely need to be made in close consultation with a healthcare provider, however, its important to offer full disclosure and inform you that discontinuation protocols are anything but settled law, they still exist in the theory phase. The decision of when and how to quit semaglutide is based on clinical acumen and an accurately painted picture of the patient, prompted by various factors, such as reaching desired weight loss goals, reaching satisfactory metabolic thresholds, experiencing intolerable side effects, or a desire to live without the medication.

Discontinuing semaglutide isn't about an abrupt stop; it's more akin to a ship gradually reducing its speed as it approaches the harbor, ensuring a controlled and smooth docking. Any overly aggressive move or missed opportunity for a smooth tapering and disaster is close behind. The tapering process typically spans several weeks, during which the dosage of semaglutide is systematically reduced, in a similar fashion to the way it was incrementally increased. This approach helps to minimize the risk of rebound weight gain and withdrawal symptoms, such as increased appetite and fluctuations in blood sugar levels. The increments are approached both in terms of dosage and time. As an example, a patient taking 1 mg per week might reduce to 0.75 mg and continue this for 4 weeks (or 4 months, depending on goals and personalized factors), then come down 0.5 mg and continue for another 4 weeks, and so on, until the medication is fully discontinued. Maybe you decide with your healthcare provider to continue with a microdosing strategy of 0.1mg per week for another year after tapering to this dose. The options are vast, which is wonderful for ideal outcomes but confusing and difficult to navigate. Throughout this process, regular monitoring of weight, blood sugar levels, and any potential side effects is crucial. This ensures that adjustments can be made as needed and helps in maintaining the gains achieved while on semaglutide.

As the dosage decreases, the focus shifts to reinforcing healthy habits and building a sustainable lifestyle. This sustainable lifestyle optimizes production and activation of natural GLP-1, which we have already well established as a powerhouse of metabolic and overall health. I have dubbed this the GLP-1 lifestyle, as you have probably noticed throughout the book thus far. This phase is critical for maintaining the benefits achieved with the medication. The GLP-1 lifestyle is powerful enough that it can be used outside of any use of semaglutide, but it is equally, or potentially more, powerful as an adjunct and a bridge from semaglutide therapy. The GLP-1 lifestyle will consume an entire section of this book, a bit later on. Transitioning from semaglutide to the GLP-1 lifestyle is not just about maintaining weight loss; it's about fostering long-term metabolic health.

Some individuals may experience a return of appetite and weight gain if not carefully managed following discontinuation of semaglutide. Careful management can mean sometimes re-adding semaglutide after discontinuation or increasing back to a dose from which side effects were reduced or unnoticeable. Feeling educated, supported and open to communicate about any issues occurring post dose reduction or discontinuation is critical, as well. The educational component should focus on the physiologic and behavioral aspects of appetite and weight management, ensuring that you understand the role of nutrition, physical activity, and psychological well-being in sustaining your weight loss.

Moreover, a gradual integration of lifestyle changes is essential to ensure new habits are sustainable and do not overwhelm the individual. This approach can significantly reduce the risk of relapse. For instance, one should feel encouraged to adopt small, manageable changes in their diet and exercise routines, progressively building up to more substantial modifications. This is exactly parallel to the "low and slow" approach taken when ramping up utilization of the medication in the first place. Nothing changes here, in fact, I would hope you are beginning to see a powerful methodology of life being presented. Rarely is it sustainable to jump full bore into a new endeavor, to go from 0% to 100% commitment overnight. The notion of mastery lies not in sporadic bursts of intensity, but in the consistent drip of daily practice. This method allows the body and mind to adjust slowly, making the transition smoother and more likely to be maintained long-term.

The science behind this gradual adaptation is rooted in neuroplasticity, the brain's remarkable ability to reorganize itself by forming new neural connections. Each "practice" session of a ramping upward or trending downward dose is like laying a brick on the path to mastery, solidifying these connections over time. The same principle applies to muscle memory, where frequent repetition etches the skill into your body's innate understanding. It is through these consistent actions, rather than infrequent marathons of effort, that habits are formed and true mastery is achieved. Tapering up and down on semaglutide is like forming a habit within your body. Embracing this approach offers psychologic benefits as well. The daunting nature of intense, infrequent dose adjustments is replaced with manageable, bite-sized chunks, reducing anxiety and fostering motivation. Witnessing incremental progress fuels the desire to continue, transforming the journey into a rewarding and enjoyable one.

Always remember, discontinuing semaglutide is part of the natural progression in your weight loss and metabolic health journey. You were never meant to stay on it forever, nor should you want to! It reflects the medication's effectiveness in jumpstarting weight loss and empowering individuals to make sustainable lifestyle changes. The transition back away from it and into your new optimal GLP-1 lifestyle is just another brick in the path of your continued journey. By approaching discontinuation with a thoughtful plan and a commitment to healthy habits, you can successfully navigate this transition and continue the voyage towards a healthier, happier life. The ultimate goal is to leverage the benefits of semaglutide while building a foundation of natural GLP-1 optimization for long-term health and well-being.

Some of you are probably wondering; what are the long term effects of semaglutide after discontinuation? It is essential to start by mentioning that our understanding is limited to initial data. These are relatively new drugs, and we do not yet fully comprehend the long-term effects. The evidence suggests that the metabolic changes induced by semaglutide are not permanent and tend to reverse after discontinuation. Studies have shown that individuals who stop taking semaglutide often experience a gradual return to their baseline metabolic state. This includes a decrease in insulin sensitivity, an increase in appetite, and a resumption of normal gastric emptying rates. The reversal of these effects can lead to weight regain and a potential worsening of blood sugar control. This sounds negative, however, it is my belief that we are seeing the effects of a first generation of users who did not fully optimize their GLP-1 lifestyle. This won't happen to you.

Not everyone experiences a complete reversal of metabolic effects after discontinuing semaglutide, many are able to maintain some of the benefits. More than likely, these individuals were particularly effective in making a shift toward a GLP-1 lifestyle. This suggests that the foundation built with healthier habits while on semaglutide can help sustain metabolic improvements once off or tapering down the medication.

The degree and duration of metabolic changes after semaglutide discontinuation can vary depending on several factors. These factors include the duration of treatment, the dose of the medication, individual differences in physiology, and the presence of other underlying health conditions. For instance, someone who has been on semaglutide for an extended period may experience different effects than someone who used the medication for a shorter duration. Additionally, individuals with better baseline metabolic health or those who have consistently engaged in lifestyle modifications may find it easier to maintain some benefits post-discontinuation. The return of appetite and normal gastric emptying rates can pose significant challenges. The increase in hunger and the return of faster digestion can lead to increased food intake, making weight maintenance difficult. Here, we can see how individualized semaglutide use dictates the approach to that steady docking of the ship. None of this is one size fits all.

The psychologic impact of discontinuing semaglutide should not be underestimated. Individuals who have experienced significant weight loss and improved metabolic health may find the prospect of reversing these gains distressing. Ensuring psychological support and counseling during this transition period can help to cope with the changes and maintain a commitment to a healthy lifestyle.

In the next section, we will dive deeper into the fascinating realm of health mastery, shifting away from a completely focused discussion on semaglutide and instead moving toward overarching ideas within the GLP-1 lifestyle. Our journey begins with the gut, often referred to as the "second brain" due to its intricate connection to overall well-being. Next, we'll venture into the intriguing world environmental health, where you will learn how your environment greatly impacts your health. Through this exploration, we'll gain a deeper appreciation for the intricate connections within our bodies and the power we have to influence our own well-being.

SECTION IV: GUT HEALTH = OVERALL HEALTH

CHAPTER 19: PROBIOTICS MATTER

Some of you may be wondering why I am introducing a deep dive into gut health in a book dedicated to semaglutide and GLP-1. The answer is twofold. First, the two are intimately linked. The goals of semaglutide use, or naturally optimizing GLP-1, align perfectly with the goals of attaining bulletproof gut health. There is strong evidence that the gut microbiome can influence hunger, cravings, metabolism, insulin sensitivity, and fat loss. Using a medication like semaglutide while ignoring gut health would be foolhardy and a waste of time and money. I promise you that within the next couple of years, it will become clear that achieving gut health and a more optimal microbiome is a critical factor in success after semaglutide use. By focusing on this now, I am offering you a key to future therapy.

No doubt you have come across gut health in the past year, it's everywhere—prebiotics, probiotics, fiber, and peptides. In the past, it has been easy to overlook the gut, hidden as it is within the depths of our abdomen. But this unassuming organ complex is far more than just a food processing plant, it's a command center, a communication hub, and a powerful influencer of our overall health. As it stands today, it is emerging as the primary influencer of overall health. The gut microbiome in particular, the collective term for the microorganisms residing in our digestive tract, is a diverse and dynamic community with far reaching health influence. It's a vast array of species, each with its own unique role to play in maintaining balance and harmony within the gut ecosystem.

The gut plays a crucial role in digestion, breaking down food, extracting nutrients, and producing essential vitamins and short-chain fatty acids. It also produces neurotransmitters and hormones that greatly influence your mood and sleep. The gut is the epicenter of the entire immune system; that common cold you couldn't avoid, the flu that stuck around a couple of weeks longer than it should have, even that unexpected cancer diagnosis—all potentially share their beginnings in the gut. And guess what? The gut produces GLP-1, therefore aiding influence over your food choices, your ability to lose weight, and your metabolism, among other aspects we've discussed.

When semaglutide enters the scene, your gut immediately undergoes a series of adjustments, but, what are semaglutide's effects on overall gut health, the microbiome, and postbiotic production? The composition of your gut's bacterial community may change, with some species thriving while others decline. Research suggests that semaglutide tends to favor the growth of beneficial bacteria that produce short-chain fatty acids (SCFAs) like butyrate. These changes can enhance gut health and contribute to improved metabolic function.

However, this microbial reshuffling can also have some downsides. In the short term, semaglutide's impact on the gut can be a bit of a mixed bag. While it offers potential benefits like improved nutrient absorption and a healthier microbiome, it can also cause the temporary discomfort and digestive upset we discussed at length. It is essential for you to understand and accept that a sudden shift within the microbiome can come with some unpleasant side effects, like upset stomach, diarrhea and other digestive woes. This reaction is common in any gut health protocol and is often secondary to something known as "die-off." Die-off occurs when harmful bacteria in the gut die and leave behind unsavory metabolites that cause gastrointestinal upset. It's like a changing of the guard in a city, with some initial unrest and adjustment as the new regime takes hold.

While the short-term effects of semaglutide on the gut are well-documented, its long-term impact remains a subject of ongoing research and debate. As with any medication, especially those that interact with complex systems like the gut microbiome, the full extent of semaglutide's influence may take years to unfold. One of the primary concerns is the potential for lasting changes to the gut microbiome. Initial shifts in bacterial composition appear beneficial, favoring the growth of helpful bacteria that, for example, produce short-chain fatty acids like butyrate. However, the long-term consequences of this alteration are not yet fully understood.

One critical area of investigation is whether the suppression of certain bacterial species could lead to unintended consequences down the line. The gut microbiome is a highly intricate ecosystem where diverse microbial communities coexist and interact in complex ways. Disrupting this balance, even with seemingly beneficial changes, could have ripple effects that are not immediately apparent. For instance, the suppression of specific bacterial species might inadvertently weaken the gut's overall resilience, making it more susceptible to infections or dysbiosis under certain conditions. Another aspect under scrutiny is whether the microbiome's delicate balance could be permanently disrupted by long-term semaglutide use. The gut is highly adaptive, and its microbial inhabitants are constantly responding to dietary, environmental, and physiological changes. However, sustained exposure to any external factor, including medications, could potentially lead to a new, stable state that differs from the pre-treatment norm. Whether this new equilibrium is beneficial, neutral, or harmful is a question that requires further exploration.

Additionally, there is concern over the long-term effects on nutrient absorption and overall gut health. While semaglutide may initially enhance the production of beneficial postbiotics like SCFAs, which support gut health and metabolism, it's unclear if these benefits are sustainable over the long haul. Chronic use of the medication could potentially alter the gut's ability to produce these compounds independently, creating a dependency on the drug to maintain optimal gut function. Moreover, there are questions about the potential systemic effects of these changes. The gut microbiome is closely linked to numerous aspects of health, therefore, alterations here could have far-reaching implications, affecting everything from inflammation levels to neurotransmitter production to the development of cancer.

In essence, while semaglutide shows promise for managing weight and blood sugar levels, its long-term impact on the gut microbiome is a complex and evolving story. As research continues, it will be crucial to monitor not just the immediate therapeutic benefits but also the broader and more enduring consequences of altering the gut's microbial landscape. In my professional opinion, the solution to this concern lies in transitioning away from prolonged use of the medication. By gradually discontinuing semaglutide and adopting a GLP-1 lifestyle, individuals can retain the benefits of the therapy while avoiding the potential short and long-term consequences of semaglutide.

There are many positives that we need to discuss to understand both semaglutide and GLP-1's effects on the gut. One such discovery is that semaglutide can increase the abundance of Akkermansia muciniphila, a bacterium associated with improved metabolic health and reduced inflammation. This peculiar microbe, considered a guardian of the gut lining, has garnered significant attention for its beneficial role in maintaining gut integrity and promoting overall health. Akkermansia thrives in the mucus layer of the gut lining, where it helps maintain the barrier between the gut environment and the bloodstream. By doing so, it plays a crucial role in preventing inflammation and metabolic endotoxemia, a condition where harmful substances from the gut leak into the bloodstream, triggering systemic inflammation. This bacterium's ability to fortify the gut barrier is just one aspect of its health-promoting arsenal.

Interestingly, research has shown that Akkermansia can increase the number of L-cells, those specialized intestinal cells responsible for producing GLP-1. This relationship between Akkermansia and L-cells highlights a fascinating interplay between gut bacteria and host metabolism. By nurturing the growth of Akkermansia, semaglutide indirectly boosts GLP-1 secretion, enhancing its own therapeutic effects. This creates a positive feedback loop where improved gut health and increased GLP-1 levels work synergistically to promote metabolic balance.

Akkermansia is also often referred to as the "skinny bacteria" because of its profound effects on metabolism and fat storage. Studies have demonstrated that higher levels of Akkermansia are associated with a leaner physique and better metabolic profiles. This bacterium appears to influence fat storage and energy expenditure, potentially making it a key player in weight management and obesity prevention. Furthermore, Akkermansia has been linked to improved insulin sensitivity and reduced inflammation, both of which are critical factors in metabolic health. By fostering a healthier gut environment, semaglutide's promotion of Akkermansia could help mitigate metabolic disorders.

Along with Akkermansia, semaglutide—and likely native GLP-1—has the ability to increase other commensal bacteria. These are the dominant groups of bacteria within the gut microbiome that promote health. Our gut population is meant to be dominated by these beneficial bacteria, which include not only Akkermansia but also Bifidobacterium spp. and Lactobacillus spp.

Bifidobacteria deserve a book of their own. They are meant to dominate our internal landscape and promote health in a myriad of incredible ways. This group of bacteria is known for its beneficial effects on gut health, including improved digestion, enhanced immune function, and reduced inflammation. These friendly microbes have been shown to increase GLP-1 secretion and improve insulin sensitivity. By fostering a thriving population of Bifidobacterium in our gut, we can further enhance GLP-1's beneficial effects on metabolism and glucose control.

In one study, individuals who consumed a diet high in prebiotics, which preferentially support the growth of Bifidobacterium, experienced improvements in both gut health and metabolic markers. These individuals reported better digestion, fewer gastrointestinal symptoms, and improved blood sugar levels. Similarly, patients with type 2 diabetes who incorporated probiotics containing Bifidobacterium into their routine saw reductions in fasting blood glucose and HbA1c levels, indicating better long-term blood sugar control.

One notable study on a specific strain, Bifidobacterium longum BB536, published in the journal *Beneficial Microbes*, delved into its effects on gut microbiota and overall health, underscoring its potential benefits in enhancing GLP-1 secretion and improving metabolic outcomes. The administration of BB536 resulted in a substantial increase in the population of beneficial bifidobacteria within the gut. This positive shift in microbiota composition was accompanied by a decrease in harmful bacteria, such as Clostridium perfringens, indicating a more balanced and healthier gut environment. Moreover, the study observed improvements in immune function markers among those receiving BB536. There was a notable increase in the production of secretory immunoglobulin A (IgA), an antibody essential for mucosal immunity, suggesting enhanced immune defense mechanisms.

These findings highlight the therapeutic potential of just one single Bifidobacterium spp. strain, not only in promoting a healthy gut microbiome but also in supporting overall immune function. Moreover, several studies have reported an increase in Bifidobacterium spp. with GLP-1 receptor agonist use. For instance, a clinical trial involving patients with obesity and type 2 diabetes demonstrated that treatment with semaglutide not only led to significant weight loss and improved glycemic control but also increased the abundance of Bifidobacterium in the gut microbiome. These findings suggest a synergistic relationship between semaglutide and Bifidobacterium, where each enhances the other's positive effects on metabolic health.

Lactobacillus spp. represents another significant group of commensal bacteria that aid in optimizing gut health. These, too, can flourish with the use of semaglutide, highlighting the intricate interplay between this GLP-1 and gut microbiota. Known for their critical role in fostering a healthy gut environment, Lactobacilli offer a multitude of health benefits that extend far beyond simple digestion.

One of the primary functions of Lactobacillus bacteria is to maintain an acidic pH in the gut, which is crucial for inhibiting the growth of harmful pathogens. By producing lactic acid (hence their name) and other metabolites, these bacteria create an environment that is hostile to pathogenic bacteria, thereby preventing infections and promoting overall gut health. The acidic environment facilitated by Lactobacilli is essential for supporting gut barrier function, which helps to keep the gut lining intact and prevents the leakage of harmful substances into the bloodstream —a condition often referred to as "leaky gut." Moreover, Lactobacilli play a significant role in modulating the immune system. They are involved in the production of various antimicrobial peptides and other immune-modulating compounds that help to balance the immune response. This can be particularly beneficial in preventing chronic inflammation, a common underlying factor in many metabolic disorders.

Research has shown that increasing the population of Lactobacillus in the gut can have a profound impact on GLP-1 secretion. For instance, studies have indicated that these bacteria can stimulate the production of GLP-1 by enhancing the function of those same L-cells in the intestines. This in turn benefits GLP-1 production and metabolic health. Beyond these metabolic benefits, Lactobacillus bacteria also support the overall health of the gut microbiome. They compete with harmful bacteria for resources and space, thereby maintaining a balanced microbial ecosystem.

A compelling study on Lactobacillus rhamnosus GG, published in the *Journal of Clinical Gastroenterology*, provides a vivid illustration of this bacteria's profound impact on gut health and metabolic outcomes. The study's findings were striking and multifaceted. Those who took Lactobacillus rhamnosus GG experienced a significant improvement in their gut microbiota composition. There was a notable increase in the population of beneficial bacteria, including other Lactobacillus species and Bifidobacterium, while harmful bacteria such as Clostridium species were markedly reduced. This shift towards a healthier microbial balance was accompanied by several positive health outcomes.

One of the most significant findings was the enhancement of gut barrier function. Participants in the Lactobacillus group showed a marked reduction in intestinal permeability, the leaky gut referenced earlier. This improvement was evidenced by decreased levels of endotoxins in the bloodstream, indicating that fewer harmful substances were leaking from the gut into the body. The strengthened gut barrier not only reduced inflammation but also improved overall immune function. The metabolic benefits were equally impressive. Participants who received Lactobacillus rhamnosus GG demonstrated improved insulin sensitivity and better glycemic control. The study reported lower fasting blood glucose levels and a significant reduction in HbA1c. These improvements were attributed in part to the enhanced GLP-1 secretion stimulated by Lactobacillus rhamnosus GG. The bacteria's metabolites, including lactic acid, played a key role in activating the L-cells in the gut to produce more GLP-1, thus improving glucose metabolism and promoting satiety.

Moreover, the study highlighted the impact of Lactobacillus rhamnosus GG on weight management. Participants in the probiotic group experienced a significant reduction in body weight and body mass index (BMI) compared to the placebo group. This weight loss was largely attributed to the increased feeling of fullness and reduced appetite, potentially brought about by higher GLP-1 levels. The participants reported fewer cravings for high-calorie foods and a greater preference for healthier options, showcasing the potential of Lactobacillus rhamnosus GG in aiding sustainable weight loss. Also, showcasing the potential of the GLP-1 lifestyle to have a significant effect on weight loss and metabolic health.

Additionally, the anti-inflammatory effects of Lactobacillus rhamnosus GG were noteworthy. The study observed a significant decrease in markers of systemic inflammation, such as C-reactive protein (CRP) and pro-inflammatory cytokines. This reduction in inflammation is crucial for preventing the chronic diseases associated with metabolic syndrome and promoting overall health. This story of Lactobacillus rhamnosus GG exemplifies the profound impact that probiotics can have on our health.

Another fascinating study took place with Lactobacillus gasseri BNR17, published in the *Journal of Nutritional Science*, which highlights this probiotic's potential impact on visceral fat reduction. As we learned previously, visceral fat is highly malignant and can ruin one's metabolic health. The results of this study were impressive. Participants who took Lactobacillus gasseri BNR17 experienced a significant and preferential reduction in visceral fat..

On average, the probiotic group saw a reduction of visceral fat by approximately 8.5%, compared to a negligible change in the placebo group. This reduction in visceral fat was accompanied by notable improvements in several metabolic parameters. Participants in the probiotic group exhibited a significant decrease in waist circumference and body mass index (BMI), indicating overall fat loss and improved body composition. Additionally, the probiotic group showed improved insulin sensitivity and lower fasting blood glucose levels.

Lactobacillus gasseri BNR17 has been shown to reduce inflammation in the body. The study observed lower levels of inflammatory markers in this probiotic group, as well. This effect is vital for improving overall health as chronic inflammation is a surefire way to destroy any potential at an optimized existence. It is akin to a wildfire raging throughout your body, with all potential healing and health resources being used at the scene, versus elsewhere in the body.

Thats just a few of a whole host of evidence demonstrating the various ways that beneficial bacteria like Akkermansia, Bifidobacterium and Lactobacilli can support weight management and overall health through an optimization of gut health and enhancement of hormones such as GLP-1. It's the GLP-1 lifestyle at work again! Is this starting to blow your mind yet? There are so many connections, waypoints and interconnected networks pointing to and fro from gut health, mental health, healthy weight loss and overall long term health-span. Many of these networks run straight through GLP-1.

Just as promoting beneficial strains and species within our microbiome is crucial for our health, equally important is the reduction or elimination of harmful bacteria that reside in the gut. Remarkably, semaglutide use and GLP-1 optimization not only enhance the presence of beneficial bacteria but also work to diminish the population of detrimental bacteria. The significance of reducing harmful bacteria cannot be overstated. These pathogenic microorganisms can disrupt the delicate equilibrium of the gut ecosystem, leading to various health issues. For instance, bacteria such as Clostridium difficile, Escherichia coli, and certain strains of Streptococcus are known to cause infections, inflammation, and other gastrointestinal problems. By decreasing these harmful bacteria, we can prevent a range of health complications and support a more robust immune system.

Numerous studies have shown that the reduction of harmful bacteria coincides with improved metabolic outcomes, reduced inflammation, and enhanced overall health. In the broader context of health and disease prevention, the importance of maintaining a balanced gut microbiome becomes even more apparent. It appears that reducing bad bacteria has an equal effect to increasing good bacteria, and of course we know that increasing good bacteria helps to shift the equation toward even more good bacteria. It is easy to imagine the power that can come with completely re-balancing one's microbiome. This is super exciting, cutting edge and in my opinion will change the face of medicine within the next decade. A healthy gut microbiome plays a critical role in protecting against a range of conditions, including obesity, diabetes, cardiovascular diseases, and autoimmune disorders.

Among the vast cast of characters in the gut microbiome, Firmicutes emerges as a villain. It is not that we want to eliminate Firmicutes entirely (or any of the following species), but we need to keep their numbers considerably lower than those of the commensal species. Balance is key in all aspects of life, and this holds true for our gut microbiome as well. The correct balance of the following bacterial species is meant to remain quite low comparatively. Firmicutes are often more abundant in individuals with obesity and metabolic disorders. Research has highlighted a strong correlation between a high Firmicutes ratio and increased body weight. A lower abundance of Firmicutes has been associated with reduced inflammation and improved insulin sensitivity.

In a pivotal study published in *Nature*, researchers found that individuals with a higher ratio of Firmicutes in their gut microbiome were more likely to suffer from obesity. This study involved analyzing the gut microbiota of obese and lean twins, revealing that obese individuals had a higher proportion of Firmicutes compared to their lean counterparts. To further understand this, researchers conducted an experiment where they transplanted gut bacteria from obese mice into germ-free mice. The recipients of the Firmicutes dominated microbiota gained more fat than those transplanted with other species, even when consuming the same diet. This imbalance is thought to contribute to the efficiency with which these bacteria extract energy from food, leading to higher calorie absorption and, consequently, weight gain.

This is an amazing concept. Let's look at an example, Bacteroides spp. This is a genus of bacteria particularly known for its ability to break down complex carbohydrates. These bacteria are highly efficient at converting dietary fibers, resistant starches, and polysaccharides into simpler molecules that the human body can absorb and use for energy. This enhanced breakdown of carbohydrates not only aids in digestion but also increases the caloric yield from food. This means an individual who just happens to have a higher percentage of bacteroides in their guts actually absorbs more calories from every bite of food. The ancient survival benefits of this are obvious, however, elevated Bacteroides is a huge disadvantage. Thus, understanding and managing the activity of specific species that are active in macronutrient extraction is another crucial element for maintaining a healthy weight and optimizing metabolic health.

Recent studies have highlighted a potential link between an increased abundance of Firmicutes in the gut microbiome and the development of colorectal cancer. For instance, a study published in the journal *Cancer Research* found that a higher ratio of Firmicutes was associated with an increased risk of colorectal cancer. The study involved analyzing the gut microbiota composition of patients with colorectal cancer and comparing it to that of healthy controls. The researchers discovered that the patients with cancer had a significantly higher presence of Firmicutes. The study concluded that microbial dysbiosis, in this case characterized by an overrepresentation of Firmicutes, could contribute to the initiation and progression of colorectal cancer by altering the gut's metabolic environment and immune responses.

Managing levels of specific bacterial species is part of a larger strategy to optimize the gut microbiome, and an advanced one at that. Alongside promoting beneficial bacteria like Akkermansia, Bifidobacterium, and Lactobacillus, reducing the abundance of potentially harmful bacteria is ever important. This is the GLP-1 lifestyle at work, and semaglutide use can play an important role in the re-balancing act.

Streptococcus, a genus of bacteria commonly found in the oral cavity and throat, can sometimes make its way into the gut, where it becomes a less welcome guest. While many species of Streptococcus are harmless or even beneficial in their native environments, their presence in the gut can lead to an imbalance, contributing to inflammation and other health issues. Some species of Streptococcus, particularly those typically found in the oral cavity, have been linked to inflammation and gut dysbiosis. When these oral Streptococcus species make their way into the gut, they can disrupt the delicate balance of the microbiome, potentially leading to a cascade of negative health consequences. It is important for you to understand that these normal oral microbes would never make their way into the gut if a healthy microbiome and state of metabolic health existed in the host human. This is the link that much of medicine is missing.

Studies have shown that an overabundance of Streptococcus in the gut can trigger inflammation, impair gut barrier function, and contribute to the development of chronic diseases like inflammatory bowel disease (IBD) and even cardiovascular disease. This is largely due to the inflammatory nature of some Streptococcus species, which can produce metabolites that irritate the gut lining and provoke an immune response. This inflammation can damage the gut barrier, allowing harmful substances to leak into the bloodstream, the leaky gut syndrome that I have mentioned a few times now.

A study published in *Gastroenterology* investigated the relationship between Streptococcus overgrowth in the gut and chronic inflammation. Researchers analyzed the gut microbiota of patients with inflammatory bowel disease (IBD) and found a significantly higher abundance of Streptococcus species compared to healthy controls. This overrepresentation of Streptococcus was associated with increased levels of pro-inflammatory cytokines, which are signaling molecules that can exacerbate inflammation.

Once in the bloodstream, these harmful substances can trigger systemic inflammation, which is a risk factor for a range of chronic conditions, including IBD and cardiovascular disease. The presence of Streptococcus in the gut is particularly concerning because these bacteria are adept at forming biofilms, which are protective layers that shield them from the immune system and antibiotics. This makes them difficult to eradicate once they establish a foothold in the gut.

To further understand the impact of Streptococcus on gut health, researchers conducted an experiment on mice. They introduced a high number of Streptococcus bacteria into the guts of germ-free mice, which led to the development of gut inflammation and impaired gut barrier function. The study concluded that an overgrowth of Streptococcus could disrupt the delicate balance of the gut microbiome, triggering inflammation and contributing to the progression of disease.

The microbial remodeling observed with semaglutide use is not merely a side effect of the medication; it's likely an integral part of its therapeutic mechanism. In other words, GLP-1's effects on the gut are likely a primary mechanism contributing to its effectiveness for weight management. This makes perfect sense, given that the gut microbiome plays a crucial role in appetite regulation, glucose metabolism, and energy balance. By altering the composition of the microbiome, semaglutide may influence these processes, thereby contributing to its effects on weight loss and blood sugar control.

Furthermore, changes in the gut microbiome induced by semaglutide may have long-term implications for gut health and overall well-being. A healthier, more balanced gut microbiome can enhance nutrient absorption, reduce inflammation, and support immune function, creating a positive feedback loop that reinforces the benefits. By nurturing a thriving population of beneficial bacteria and suppressing harmful ones, semaglutide not only aids in immediate weight loss and glycemic control but also sets the stage for sustained health improvements.

As we conclude this chapter on probiotics, it becomes evident that these microscopic allies play a monumental role in maintaining and enhancing our health. Probiotics, particularly the beneficial strains like Bifidobacterium and Lactobacillus, are crucial for fostering a balanced and resilient gut. Through their various mechanisms, they support digestion, strengthen the barrier, modulate the immune system, and greatly influence metabolic health.

The studies we've explored illustrate the profound impact of specific probiotic strains. From Bifidobacterium BB536 aiding in digestion and immunity to Lactobacillus gasseri BNR17 helping to reduce visceral fat, the evidence is clear: fostering a healthy gut microbiome is a cornerstone of metabolic health and disease prevention.

As research continues to unfold, the potential for probiotics in preventive and therapeutic health strategies will undoubtedly expand. By incorporating probiotics into our daily lives, we not only support our gut health but also enhance our overall vitality and resilience. The journey towards optimal health is a multifaceted one, and probiotics are indispensable companions on this path.

CHAPTER 20: PREBIOTICS PROBABLY MATTER MORE

These are not just the hottest trend of the last two years or the newest, necessary ingredient in any protein shake formulation. Prebiotics are absolutely essential; the non-digestible fibers that travel to the lower gut, where they act as food for the microbiome, stimulating the growth and activity of beneficial bacteria.

Prebiotics work by selectively stimulating the growth and activity of beneficial bacteria, the commensal species we discussed in the previous chapter. This selective feeding mechanism is crucial because it ensures that the most helpful bacterial species thrive. These fibers, which our bodies cannot digest, travel through the upper parts of the gastrointestinal tract unchanged until they reach the colon. Via the beneficial bacteria, these fibers undergo fermentation in the lower gut, which allows for the production of postbiotics, an emerging field that demonstrates incredible potential.

Alongside feeding the growth of beneficial bacteria, prebiotics also aid in the digestion and absorption of nutrients, better equipping the host (you) to break down complex carbohydrates, proteins, and fats. This ensures that the body gets the maximum nutritional benefit and caloric delivery from food. Prebiotics have been shown to improve the absorption of minerals such as calcium and magnesium, expanding their role to bone health, muscle health, athletic performance and a myriad of physiologic processes. Prebiotics help to support the gut-associated lymphoid tissue

(GALT), which plays a key role in building the immune system as a whole.

Prebiotics come in various forms, each with unique properties and benefits, and they are naturally found in a variety of foods and can also be taken as dietary supplements. The amazing thing is that incorporating prebiotics into your diet is a natural and effective way to support health and enhance the activity of beneficial bacteria, while offering essentially zero downsides. Foods such as garlic, onions, leeks, asparagus, bananas, and whole grains are excellent sources of prebiotics and can easily be included in daily meals.

Inulin is one of the most well-known and widely studied prebiotics. Found in plants like chicory root, garlic, onions, leeks, asparagus, Jerusalem artichokes, and bananas, inulin is particularly effective at stimulating the growth of beneficial bacteria like Bifidobacterium and Lactobacillus. Its benefits include enhanced digestion, improved nutrient absorption, better immune function, and regulated blood sugar levels.

Fructooligosaccharides (FOS), similar to inulin, are short-chain fructose molecules that promote the growth of beneficial gut bacteria. These are found in garlic, onions, leeks, asparagus, bananas, blue agave, and yacon root, and they help enhance immune function, improve bowel regularity, and support healthy cholesterol levels.

Galactooligosaccharides (GOS) are another type of prebiotic fiber composed of galactose molecules, particularly beneficial for Bifidobacterium species. Found in legumes and certain vegetables like beets and artichokes, GOS supports gut health and immune function, reduces infection risk, and may alleviate symptoms of irritable bowel syndrome (IBS).

Arabinogalactans, complex polysaccharides from arabinose and galactose molecules, are found in larch trees, carrots, radishes, pears, tomatoes, and corn. These fibers stimulate the growth of beneficial gut bacteria, support immune function, and may improve gut barrier function and reduce inflammation.

Pectin, a soluble fiber in the cell walls of fruits like apples, citrus, berries, peaches, plums, and carrots, forms a gel-like substance in the gut, aiding digestion and promoting the growth of beneficial bacteria. It helps regulate bowel movements, reduce cholesterol levels, and control blood sugar.

Resistant starch (RS), which resists digestion in the small intestine and ferments in the large intestine, is found in unripe bananas, cooked and cooled potatoes, rice, pasta, whole grains, and legumes. RS is particularly potent and very important to begin incorporating into your diet. It greatly promotes beneficial gut bacteria, seals the gut barrier, enhances insulin sensitivity, and aids in weight management.

Oligosaccharides, a group of prebiotics including various short-chain carbohydrates, are found in soybeans, whole grains, onions, garlic, leeks, and asparagus. They stimulate the growth of beneficial gut bacteria, support immune function, enhance mineral absorption, and may reduce the risk of colon cancer by promoting a healthy gut environment.

One of the most exciting aspects of prebiotics is their ability to enhance the production of GLP-1. The fermentation of prebiotic fibers leads to metabolic byproducts (postbiotics) that can stimulate the release of GLP-1 from the intestinal L-cells. This is only one single benefit of prebiotic consumption, however, you are already aware of the far reaching benefits.

There are trends occurring in today's eating patterns which are moving away from the consumption of plant foods and prebiotics. These diets, often touted for their immediate benefits and improvements in well-being, have gained popularity for a reason. However, it's essential to recognize that the reason individuals feel better on these diets is almost invariably because they have non-optimized guts, nearly guaranteed to suffer from dysbiosis and likely some degree of irritable bowel syndrome (IBS) or inflammatory bowel disease (IBD).

The epidemic proportions of common GI disease like IBS, dysbiosis and leaky gut has led to a trend of people moving away from plant foods. As our modern diets have increasingly favored processed foods, convenience foods, pesticides and chemicals, the overall health of our guts has deteriorated. This has resulted in weaker gut health, making it more challenging for some to digest and tolerate the high-fiber content found in many prebiotic-rich plant foods. Consequently, individuals may find themselves in a catch-22 situation, needing prebiotics to improve gut health but struggling with the temporary discomfort they can cause.

When an individual with poor gut health consumes plant fibers, the harmful bacteria in their gut produce metabolites that cause gastrointestinal distress. These harmful byproducts can lead to discomfort, such as bloating, gas, and cramping. Additionally, gut systems that are not accustomed to a high fiber load are likely to experience significant bloating and gas, secondary to the fermentation of these fibers by the microbiome, good gut bacteria included. This can create a negative feedback loop, where individuals avoid high-fiber foods to prevent discomfort, further depriving their gut microbiome of the essential nutrients it needs to thrive. This is a notable strategy in such diets as FODMAP and carnivore.

However, this avoidance strategy is not a sustainable solution. The discomfort experienced is not due to an inherent problem with plant foods, but rather a reflection of an imbalanced gut microbiome. The long-term solution lies in gradually reintroducing a lifestyle that aids the proliferation of beneficial bacteria, which will promote overall healing of the gut. Over time, this approach can restore balance to the gut microbiome, reducing symptoms of dysbiosis and IBS, and ultimately leading to improved overall health.

By understanding the root cause of this discomfort and addressing it through a gradual and mindful approach to diet, individuals can overcome these challenges. Prebiotics play a crucial role in this process, helping to feed and nurture beneficial gut bacteria, promoting a healthier and more resilient digestive system.

Incorporating prebiotics into your diet is very easy. Most plant foods contain a variety of prebiotics. Legumes and grains are loaded with prebiotic fibers. Supplements offer a convenient alternative and means to incorporate a large amount of fiber in the diet, look for inulin, green banana flour, potato starch or acacia fiber. However, it is important to approach prebiotic supplementation with care, starting with lower doses to avoid gastrointestinal discomfort. We will discuss these strategies in detail in the next section of the book.

CHAPTER 21: POSTBIOTICS MIGHT MATTER MOST

Emerging research will continue to reveal the power the gut has over our overall health. One fascinating example is the concept of postbiotics, a term that has only recently gained popularity but holds incredible potential for positive health outcomes. Postbiotics are the byproducts of the microbiome's metabolic activities. These are the molecular remnants left behind after bacteria have feasted on dietary fiber and other nutrients. Think of postbiotics as the exhaust fumes of the gut's microscopic factories. But unlike the noxious fumes of industrial processes, these byproducts are often beneficial; acting as signaling molecules, energy sources, and even weapons against harmful microbes. It is all too likely the health benefits of probiotics as we know them are primarily due to the postbiotic metabolites these beneficial bacteria produce.

This would make postbiotics the unsung heroes of the gut, working tirelessly behind the scenes to maintain balance and promote health. They function as vital communication signals between the gut microbiome and the host, influencing metabolic pathways, modulating the immune response, and even impacting mental health through the gut-brain axis. As research continues to uncover the diverse roles of postbiotics, their significance in our quest for optimal health becomes increasingly apparent. Understanding the profound impact of these byproducts aligns with the goals of semaglutide use or naturally optimized GLP-1 levels. By focusing on gut health, we can leverage these insights to enhance our overall well-being, making informed choices that support both metabolic health and long-term vitality.

For instance, take the production of bacteriocins as byproducts within the microbiome. Bacteriocins are antimicrobial peptides that inhibit the growth of harmful bacteria, thereby maintaining a balanced microbial community in the gut. Therefore, the postbiotics from beneficial bacteria are creating a positive feedback cycle for the production of more beneficial bacteria. Amazing stuff!

Another example are the short-chain fatty acids (SCFAs), a type of postbiotic produced when gut bacteria ferment fiber. SCFAs, such as butyrate, acetate, and propionate, play crucial roles in maintaining gut health and supporting the immune system. They are like the fuel that powers the gut's intricate machinery, providing energy for the cells lining the colon and keeping them healthy. However, their influence extends far beyond the gut. SCFAs reduce inflammation by inhibiting the production of pro-inflammatory cytokines and promoting the release of anti-inflammatory molecules. This anti-inflammatory effect extends beyond the gut, impacting systemic inflammation that can contribute to chronic diseases such as cardiovascular disease, diabetes, and autoimmune disorders. For instance, butyrate has been found to suppress nuclear factor-kappa B (NF-κB), a key regulator of inflammation, thereby reducing inflammatory responses throughout the body.

In addition to their anti-inflammatory properties, SCFAs play a crucial role in strengthening the gut barrier. Butyrate, in particular, is essential for maintaining the integrity of the tight junctions between intestinal cells. By enhancing the expression of tight junction proteins, butyrate helps to seal the gut lining, preventing the leaky gut phenomenon that is associated with various health issues, including autoimmune diseases and metabolic disorders.

SCFAs also influence appetite and blood sugar regulation, acting as tiny messengers that communicate with various organs and systems in the body and I bet by now, you can guess the mechanism. Butyrate and other SCFAs can stimulate the release of GLP-1 and peptide YY (PYY)! This means that there is significant synergistic potential between not just semaglutide and butyrate, but a GLP-1 lifestyle and overall gut health. Moreover, SCFAs improve insulin sensitivity and enhance glucose uptake within cells, contributing to better blood sugar control. Whether this is secondary to stimulation of GLP-1 or SCFAs functioning as a primary mechanism isn't entirely clear.

Butyrate is the most famous SCFA and the one you may have heard of, studies have shown that it plays a crucial role in preventing and managing various health conditions. In inflammatory bowel disease (IBD), for example, butyrate has been shown to reduce inflammation and promote healing of the gut lining. We will discuss these diseases as well as Irritable Bowel Syndrome (IBS) later in the book. In colon cancer, butyrate may inhibit the growth of cancer cells and promote their death. And in obesity and type 2 diabetes, butyrate may improve insulin sensitivity and glucose metabolism, potentially aiding in weight loss and blood sugar control.

Acetate, another SCFA produced by the fermentation of prebiotics, also contributes to gut health by acting as a signaling molecule that influences appetite regulation and metabolic processes. Acetate has been shown to stimulate the release of GLP-1, enhancing its beneficial effects on blood sugar control and appetite suppression.

Propionate, the third major SCFA, has been linked to improved glucose metabolism and reduced fat storage. It works by influencing pathways involved in insulin sensitivity and energy expenditure, thereby supporting metabolic health. Propionate's role in reducing liver fat accumulation is particularly important for preventing conditions like non-alcoholic fatty liver disease (NAFLD), which is heavily correlated with obesity and metabolic syndrome.

Vitamins are also part of the postbiotic arsenal produced by our gut microbiome. The gut microbiome acts as a master chemist, capable of synthesizing vitamin K and several B vitamins. These vitamins are crucial for a wide array of physiological functions, from blood clotting and energy production to nerve function and overall health. A healthy gut microbiome, rich in diverse bacteria, functions like a well-oiled vitamin factory, ensuring a steady supply of these vital nutrients. In fact, within postbiotics, we have likely discovered why so many individuals are vitamin and micronutrient deficient.

Vitamin K is essential for blood clotting and bone health, among other roles. The gut microbiome produces vitamin K2, which plays a crucial role in the regulation of calcium, thereby supporting cardiovascular health by preventing calcification of arteries and veins. This vitamin is indispensable for maintaining strong bones and facilitating proper wound healing. In fact, one of the pioneers of health described it as a super-factor for wellness. Weston A. Price, a dentist and nutrition researcher in the early 20th century, traveled the world studying the diets and health of isolated populations. He observed that people who consumed traditional diets were remarkably free from dental decay and chronic diseases.

One of his most intriguing discoveries came in the Swiss Alps, where Price studied the robust villagers who consumed raw milk, cheese, and butter from grass-fed cows. He noticed that these foods were rich in what he coined "Activator X", a substance that seemed to confer extraordinary health benefits, particularly in dental health and bone structure. Similarly, in the outer Hebrides, he found that the local diet, rich in fish and fish organs, also contained high levels of this elusive nutrient. It wasn't until decades later that researchers identified this X factor as vitamin K2. Vitamin K2, particularly in its forms produced by grass-fed animals and fermented foods, was found to direct calcium to the bones and teeth, where it is needed, and away from the cardiovascular system, where it is most unwelcome. This revelation linked Price's observations with modern nutritional science, demonstrating how traditional diets were naturally rich in vitamin K2. The villagers' strong teeth and bones, and their resistance to chronic disease, were due, in part, to the ample amounts of K2 in their diets. This nutrient synergy underscores the profound connection between diet, gut optimization and health. Optimizing our microbiome to enhance the production of vitamin K2 can bring us closer to these traditional dietary benefits.

B vitamins, synthesized by gut bacteria, are equally vital. This complex of vitamins includes B1 (thiamine), B2 (riboflavin), B3 (niacin), B5 (pantothenic acid), B6 (pyridoxine), B7 (biotin), B9 (folate), and B12 (cobalamin). Each of these vitamins plays a specific role in maintaining health. The interplay between consuming B vitamins through diet and their production by gut bacteria is a fascinating and complex relationship. Dietary intake of B vitamins provides a direct and reliable source, ensuring that the body receives these essential nutrients necessary for various physiological functions. Foods such as leafy greens, nuts, seeds, meats, and dairy products offer a spectrum of B vitamins that support the body's broad nutritional needs. This variety and balance are crucial. However, given the deteriorated health of our modern guts and our overall vitamin deficiencies, it is likely that the microbiome's role in B vitamin production is meant to supersede that of dietary intake. Historically, humans likely obtained a substantial portion of their B vitamins from gut production, supported by a fiber-rich diet that promoted a diverse and healthy microbiome.

Vitamin B1, or thiamine, is crucial for energy metabolism and nerve function. It acts as a coenzyme in the catabolic pathway of carbohydrates, playing a key role in converting nutrients into energy. Specifically, thiamine is involved in the Krebs cycle, a series of chemical reactions used by all aerobic organisms to generate energy. By facilitating the conversion of glucose into ATP (adenosine triphosphate), the primary energy currency of cells, thiamine ensures that cells have the energy they need to function properly. Moreover, thiamine is essential for the metabolic pathways involved in efficient glucose metabolism. Thiamine also plays a significant role in nerve function. It is involved in the synthesis of neurotransmitters, the chemical messengers that transmit signals across nerve cells. This is vital for maintaining healthy nerve function and supporting the communication pathways between the brain and the digestive system, including the regulation of gut motility and the release of hormones like GLP-1. The implications of all of this to metabolic health are crystal clear, I hope.

Vitamin B2, or riboflavin, is a water-soluble vitamin that plays a pivotal role in several metabolic processes essential for maintaining overall health. One of its primary functions is in energy production. Riboflavin is a crucial component of two major coenzymes involved in redox reactions within the mitochondria, the energy powerhouses of the cell. They are integral to the electron transport chain, where they facilitate the conversion of nutrients into ATP. In addition, riboflavin is essential for the metabolism of fats, drugs, and steroids. It acts as a coenzyme in the beta-oxidation of fatty acids, a process by which fatty acids are broken down to generate acetyl-CoA for energy production. This is crucial for maintaining lipid balance. Riboflavin also plays a role in detoxification processes in the liver, where it aids in the metabolism of various drugs and steroids, helping to convert them into more water-soluble forms that can be excreted from the body. Another significant function of riboflavin is its involvement in the conversion of other B vitamins into their active forms. For example, it is required for the conversion of vitamin B6 (pyridoxine) to its active form and the conversion of tryptophan to niacin (vitamin B3).

Vitamin B3, or niacin, is a vital nutrient with a wide array of roles in the body, contributing to numerous physiologic processes that are crucial for maintaining health. One of the primary functions of niacin is its role in DNA repair and the production of stress and sex hormones. Niacin is a precursor to the coenzymes nicotinamide adenine dinucleotide (NAD) and nicotinamide adenine dinucleotide phosphate (NADP), which are essential for redox reactions in the body. These coenzymes are involved in more than 400 enzymatic reactions, making niacin indispensable for energy metabolism, cell signaling, and DNA repair processes.

Just look at how much money people are spending on NAD intravenous injections these days!

DNA repair is critical for maintaining the integrity of the genetic material and preventing mutations that could lead to cancer and other diseases. NAD+ plays a crucial role in this process by participating in the repair of single-strand DNA breaks through special enzymes that detect and signal DNA damage. Niacin is also involved in the synthesis of steroid hormones, including stress hormones like cortisol and sex hormones such as testosterone and estrogen. These hormones are derived from cholesterol and require NADPH. Additionally, niacin plays a significant role in improving cholesterol levels and supporting cardiovascular health. It has been shown to increase high-density lipoprotein (HDL) cholesterol, which helps remove low-density lipoprotein (LDL) cholesterol from the bloodstream, thereby reducing the risk of atherosclerosis and cardiovascular diseases. Niacin also lowers triglyceride levels and reduces the production of very-low-density lipoprotein (VLDL) cholesterol in the liver, further contributing to a healthier lipid profile. Niacin also enhances the barrier function of the skin, protecting against environmental damage, and helps retain moisture, thereby preventing dryness and irritation. Niacin also has anti-inflammatory properties that can benefit conditions like acne, rosacea, and other inflammatory skin disorders. Quite an impressive list!

Vitamin B5, or pantothenic acid, is a water-soluble vitamin that plays a crucial role in various metabolic processes essential for maintaining overall health. One of its primary functions is the synthesis of coenzyme A (CoA), a pivotal molecule in the metabolism of fatty acids. Coenzyme A is a cofactor involved in the enzymatic reactions that catalyze the breakdown and synthesis of fatty acids, facilitating their conversion into usable energy. Coenzyme A is also integral to the Krebs cycle, that series of chemical reactions that generate ATP. Through this, CoA aids in the conversion of carbohydrates, fats, and proteins into energy. Without adequate pantothenic acid, the synthesis of CoA would be compromised, leading to impaired energy production and metabolic inefficiency. Pantothenic acid also plays a significant role in the production of red blood cells. It is involved in the synthesis of heme, which is responsible for oxygen transport in the blood. Adequate levels of pantothenic acid ensure efficient oxygen delivery to tissues. Additionally, pantothenic acid contributes to the synthesis of neurotransmitters, steroid hormones, and vitamins such as vitamin D. It is involved in the production of acetylcholine, a neurotransmitter essential for communication between nerve cells, muscle contraction, and various brain functions.

Vitamin B6, also known as pyridoxine, is a versatile and essential nutrient that plays a critical role in numerous physiologic processes. One of its primary functions is as a coenzyme for a variety of enzymes involved in the metabolism of amino acids, which are the building blocks of proteins. Neurotransmitter synthesis is another crucial role of vitamin B6. It is a cofactor for the enzymes that synthesize neurotransmitters such as serotonin, dopamine, gamma-aminobutyric acid (GABA), and norepinephrine. These neurotransmitters are essential for regulating mood, cognition, and nervous system function. In addition to its roles in amino acid metabolism and neurotransmitter synthesis, vitamin B6 participates in the regulation of gene expression by acting as a cofactor for enzymes involved in DNA methylation and histone modification. These processes are essential for controlling which genes are turned on or off in response to various physiologic and environmental signals. Vitamin B6 is also vital for the production of hemoglobin, the protein in red blood cells that carries oxygen from the lungs to the tissues and returns carbon dioxide from the tissues to the lungs. Vitamin B6 is a multifaceted nutrient that plays essential roles that contribute to overall health and well-being.

Vitamin B7, commonly known as biotin, has primary roles in the metabolism of carbohydrates and fats. As a coenzyme, biotin is essential for the function of key steps within metabolic pathways, including the synthesis and breakdown of fatty acids and metabolism of certain amino acids. Biotin is also a critical cofactor in the metabolic pathway that generates glucose from non-carbohydrate substrates, making it critical in states of fasting. The impact of biotin on skin, hair, and nail health is well-documented. Biotin is essential for the maintenance of keratin infrastructure and adequate levels of biotin contribute to the strength and resilience of these tissues. Moreover, biotin's effects on fatty acids support the skin barrier and overall skin health as well as nail and hair health.

Vitamin B9, commonly known as folate, is an essential nutrient that plays a pivotal role in DNA synthesis and repair, making it especially vital during periods of rapid growth and development, such as pregnancy and fetal development. Folate acts as a coenzyme for the building blocks of DNA, which are crucial for cell division and the formation of new cells. This is why proper levels of folate are so critical during fetal development. Beyond its role in pregnancy, folate is essential for the methylation cycle which controls gene expression, protein function, and neurotransmitter synthesis. This influences detoxification, immune response, and mood regulation.

Vitamin B12, or cobalamin, plays a crucial role in maintaining neurologic function, DNA synthesis, and red blood cell production. Vitamin B12 is involved in the synthesis of the protective sheath that surrounds nerve fibers, which is crucial for the efficient transmission of nerve impulses throughout the body. Vitamin B12 also plays a key role in red blood cell production and is necessary for the proper maturation of red blood cells in the bone marrow. The consequences of vitamin B12 deficiency are severe and multifaceted. Besides the neurological and hematological effects, chronic deficiency can also lead to elevated levels of homocysteine, an amino acid linked to an increased risk of cardiovascular diseases.

As you can clearly see, vitamins produced by the microbiome are essential for numerous physiologic functions and overall metabolic health. These vitamins play critical roles in energy production, DNA synthesis, nerve function, red blood cell formation and cardiovascular health, to name a few. The microbiome's ability to synthesize these vitamins highlights the intricate relationship between gut health and overall well-being. The link is simply unavoidable.

Finally, let's discuss antimicrobial peptides (AMP), which serve as the gut's first line of defense against harmful invaders. This frontline defense is absolutely critical for immunity within the gut and has potential implications for all chronic disease and cancer states. These small proteins, produced by certain bacteria and host cells, play a crucial role in maintaining the health and integrity of the gut microbiome. AMPs have potent antimicrobial properties, capable of killing or inhibiting the growth of a wide range of pathogens, including bacteria, viruses, and fungi. AMPs function by disrupting the cell membranes and interfering with essential cellular processes of invading pathogens.

The production of AMPs is tightly regulated by the gut's immune system, with factors such as microbiome health, diet, stress, and infection influencing levels. For instance, certain dietary components, such as fibers and polyphenols, can enhance the production of AMPs. Conversely, a diet high in processed foods and low in nutrients can impair AMP production and compromise gut immunity.

One of the most well-known classes of AMPs is defensins. Defensins are produced by epithelial cells lining the gut and have a broad spectrum of activity. Defensins not only kill pathogens directly but also recruit immune cells to sites of infection. Another important class of AMPs is cathelicidins. These peptides play a significant role in innate immunity. Cathelicidins have been shown to have antimicrobial, anti-inflammatory, and immunomodulatory properties. In the gut, they help maintain the balance of the microbiome by controlling the growth of potentially harmful bacteria while promoting the growth of beneficial ones.

AMPs also play a critical role in maintaining the barrier function of the gut lining, they contribute to this integrity by promoting the health of epithelial cells and preventing infections that could lead to inflammation and barrier disruption. This function is particularly important in conditions like leaky gut, inflammatory bowel disease (IBD) and potentially irritable bowel syndrome (IBS), any disease state where barrier integrity is often compromised.

Postbiotics are pretty amazing, aren't they? The role they play in maintaining gut health and overall metabolic function cannot be overstated. These compounds act as signaling molecules, regulate inflammation, and enhance gut barrier integrity. They support immune function, modulate blood sugar levels, are essential for energy production, blood clotting, and bone health. The importance of postbiotics lies in their ability to mediate the beneficial effects of probiotics, in fact, one must wonder; are we ultimately supporting beneficial bacteria so that we can utilize their postbiotics? This is an intriguing question and I believe in the next decade we will answer this with a resounding yes, understanding better that postbiotics regulate our metabolic, cognitive and vascular health as well as provide the base of our immunity pyramid, modulating perfectly the dance between promoting beneficial acute inflammation when needed and discouraging chronic inflammation and cancer states.

CHAPTER 22: LIVING IN A ROCKSTAR ENVIRONMENT

Our environmental exposure plays a pivotal role in shaping our health. Much like the probiotics that have promoted our health, we have relied on sunshine, water and unadulterated food for millennia. Beyond the confines of strictly defined diet and exercise, the world around us—the air we breathe, the water we drink, the sunlight we soak up, and the nature we immerse ourselves in—exerts profound influences on our physiologic and psychologic well-being. This chapter delves into the intricate interplay between our environment and health, uncovering the often-overlooked factors that can either bolster or undermine our efforts towards optimal wellness. By understanding these elements, we can create a foundation for a healthier, more vibrant life, where the benefits of taking a medication like semaglutide are fully realized and sustained.

The sun plays a pivotal role in overall health, particularly in relation to gut health, metabolic optimization, and the effects of hormones like GLP-1. Sunshine is a full spectrum of light, including perfect ratios of blue light, red light and purple light (UV light). These ratios differ throughout the day, with a dominance of red light occurring in the morning and purple light occurring in the heat of the day. The mammalian body is perfectly aligned with this daily solar rhythm, with thousands of metabolic and cellular processes being critically aligned to the position of the sun in the sky.

The emerging field of photobiomodulation (PBM) has garnered significant and deserved attention recently for its benefits in gut health and overall well-being. Put simply, this refers to affecting our bodily processes with light. Red light therapy, in particular, involves exposing the body to low levels of red or near-infrared light, which can penetrate the skin and stimulate various biological processes. This therapy has shown promise in a range of health areas, from reducing inflammation to enhancing cellular energy production. First and foremost, always keep in mind that there is no greater red light source than the one blazing above you in the sky, regardless of the time of day!

Red light therapy works by stimulating the mitochondria, the powerhouses of cells, to produce more adenosine triphosphate (ATP), the molecule responsible for energy transfer within cells. By boosting mitochondrial function, red light therapy can enhance cellular metabolism, reduce oxidative stress, and promote tissue repair and regeneration. This mechanism is particularly relevant for gut health, where efficient cellular function is crucial for maintaining the integrity of the gut lining and supporting a balanced microbiome. Research has indicated that red light therapy can reduce inflammation in the gut and promote tissue healing, alleviating symptoms stemming from IBS, IBD or any other abdominal ailment.

Moreover, red light therapy has been shown to support the growth of beneficial gut bacteria. In studies, exposure to red light has been linked to an increase in microbial diversity. The therapy's ability to enhance mitochondrial function and cellular repair can create a more favorable environment for these beneficial bacteria to thrive. By reducing systemic inflammation and oxidative stress, it can contribute to improved metabolic health, better skin conditions, enhanced muscle recovery, and even cognitive function. Regular sessions of red light therapy can even help maintain a balanced immune response.

Ultraviolet (UV) light has a profound impact on our gut health in ways that are likely familiar to you. Exposure to a specific spectrum of sunlight, known as UVB, triggers the production of vitamin D in the skin. Vitamin D, often referred to as the "sunshine vitamin," deserves a book all on its own due to its extensive and crucial roles in maintaining health. It is more accurately classified as a hormone because of its broad impact on various bodily systems. Vitamin D receptors are present throughout the gut, where they play a pivotal role in maintaining the integrity of the gut lining and promoting a healthy and diverse microbiome.

The production of vitamin D begins when UVB rays from sunlight penetrate the skin, converting 7-dehydrocholesterol to pre-vitamin D3, which then becomes active vitamin D (calcitriol) after further conversion in the liver and kidneys. In the gut, vitamin D's effects are substantial. Vitamin D receptors (VDR) are expressed in the epithelial cells lining the gut, influencing various aspects of gut health. One of the primary roles of vitamin D in the gut is to maintain the integrity of the gut lining. Adequate vitamin D levels ensure these tight junctions remain robust, preventing leaky gut syndrome. Given that gut health is deteriorating and vitamin D levels plummeting, you may now understand why you have heard so much about leaky gut syndrome in the last decade!

Moreover, vitamin D plays a crucial role in modulating the immune system. It helps regulate the activity of T cells and macrophages, which are involved in identifying and responding to harmful pathogens. By promoting a balanced immune response, vitamin D helps prevent chronic inflammation and autoimmune reactions, both of which disrupt health in a myriad of ways. The influence of vitamin D extends to the composition and diversity of the gut microbiome. Research has shown that adequate vitamin D levels are associated with a more diverse and balanced microbiome. We've added yet another layer of complexity to this cycle of the microbiome and overarching health.

Lastly, vitamin D is essential for insulin sensitivity and glucose metabolism. Deficiency has been associated with insulin resistance and increased risk of type 2 diabetes. By maintaining adequate vitamin D levels through sunlight exposure, individuals can compound the benefits of a medication like semaglutide. Or, thought of differently, given the incredible potency of vitamin D, it is likely that deficiency would lead to a significantly reduced treatment potential while using semaglutide. For this reason, vitamin D levels really should be regularly checked for anyone considering or currently taking semaglutide.

Studies have shown that maintaining adequate vitamin D levels can help reduce the severity and frequency of flare-ups in diseases of the gut, such as IBD. Vitamin D's role in modulating the immune response and maintaining gut barrier integrity is particularly beneficial in these inflammatory conditions, highlighting its therapeutic potential.

Sunlight plays a critical role in regulating circadian rhythms. Regular exposure to natural light helps synchronize these rhythms, leading to better sleep, improved mood, and more efficient metabolic function. We have already tied optimal circadian rhythms with its enhancement of GLP-1 response in a previous chapter, so you know how important this can be while striving for optimal.

Recommendations for exposure to light and PBM are relatively straight forward. First, you should be aiming to get morning sun directly into your eyes, and ideally, on your abdominal skin. UV rays do not begin to take hold until approximately 9-11 am, depending greatly on the time of year and your geographic location. Even 2 minutes of morning light on your eyes and skin have been shown to improve circadian rhythm, sleep and melatonin patterning. Next, aim to be in the afternoon sun for 20 minutes at a time, multiple times if possible. Track this with seasonal vitamin D levels. We are aiming for a level over 70, not over 40 like your doctor may tell you. If you can afford it, red light panels are a great way to get unlimited levels of red light when getting outside isn't an option. They can be used nearly limitless, but 20 minutes per day is a good goal.

Grounding, also known as earthing, involves direct physical contact with the Earth's surface. This simple practice can have profound effects on overall health, particularly in relation to gut health, metabolic optimization, and GLP-1 function. The concept of grounding centers around the notion that the Earth's surface holds a subtle electric charge, which has beneficial effects on the body when absorbed through direct contact. Grounding can positively impact gut health by reducing inflammation and improving immune function. Chronic inflammation is a common issue in gut disorders, and grounding has been shown to decrease markers of inflammation.

Our connection to the Earth might influence the composition and function of the gut microbiome. While direct scientific evidence on grounding's impact on the microbiome is still emerging, there is substantial research supporting the idea that reduced inflammation and improved stress responses can foster a healthier gut environment. Grounding has been reported to enhance mood and reduce stress levels, which indirectly benefits the microbiome by reducing stress-induced dysbiosis.

Grounding can play a role in metabolic optimization by improving sleep, reducing stress, and balancing cortisol levels. You already know that cortisol, the body's primary stress hormone, can negatively impact blood sugar levels and insulin sensitivity when chronically elevated. Grounding has been shown to normalize cortisol rhythms, leading to better metabolic health. Lower stress levels and improved sleep patterns contribute to more stable blood sugar levels and enhanced insulin sensitivity, aligning with the goals of GLP-1 receptor agonist therapy. Like sunlight, grounding can help regulate circadian rhythms. Regular contact with the Earth's surface can promote better sleep quality and a more synchronized internal clock.

Grounding is as simple as having your bare feet on the Earth; grass, sand, or soil, or being immersed in a natural body of water. It is also possible to use grounding devices, though unnecessary for most. Aim for at least 20-30 minutes of grounding each day to experience its full benefits. I have suggested this to countless individuals and have received, in turn, countless surprised reactions of the immediate calming and de-stressing effect that grounding offers.

Nature bathing, also known as forest bathing or "shinrin-yoku" in Japan, involves immersing oneself in a natural environment to enhance physical, mental, and emotional well-being. This practice has profound effects on gut health, metabolic optimization, and the efficacy of GLP-1. Immersion in nature has been shown to positively influence gut health by reducing stress and promoting a diverse and healthy microbiome. Stress reduction is a key benefit of nature bathing and you may have already put these pieces together, but sun exposure, grounding and nature connection all significantly reduce stress!

Exposure to natural environments can enhance the secretion and function of GLP-1, through mechanisms we have discussed multiple times, such as stress reduction and circadian entrainment. Interestingly, spending time in nature can expose you to a wide variety of beneficial microorganisms present in the natural environment, ones you cannot be exposed to in a sterile office environment, for example. This exposure can enhance microbial diversity in the gut and can contribute to a more robust and balanced gut ecosystem.

To maximize the benefits of nature bathing for gut health, metabolic optimization, and stress relief, simply spend time in a natural environment a few times a week. Even short visits to parks, gardens, or nature reserves can have significant benefits. Spend at least 20-30 minutes per session in nature to fully immerse yourself and reap the therapeutic effects. Longer sessions can provide even greater benefits. Pay attention to the sights, sounds, and smells around you. Involve all of your senses to enhance relaxation and stress reduction. Engage in light physical activities such as walking, hiking, or yoga while in nature.

Regular physical activity has a significant impact on health, the gut included. Exercise preferentially stimulates the growth of beneficial bacteria, such as Bifidobacterium and Lactobacillus species. Studies have shown that exercise can increase microbial diversity, leading to a more resilient gut ecosystem. Physical activity promotes a balanced microbiome by enhancing gut motility and reducing the risk of dysbiosis. Exercise increases the production of SCFAs, particularly butyrate, keeping that all important gut barrier healthy and functioning. Moreover, exercise can also help manage stress and optimize mitochondria.

Metabolic health is greatly influenced by regular physical activity. Exercise enhances insulin sensitivity, allowing cells to more effectively take up glucose for energy. This reduces blood sugar levels, improves metabolic health and aids with the effectiveness of semaglutide. Physical activity also increases energy expenditure, in a couple of ways. First, of course, the act of moving burns calories and increases expenditure directly. However, more importantly, exercise builds muscle and muscle is a metabolic organ, as we discussed previously. Individuals with more muscle mass burn more calories at rest, this is an unfair advantage you should consider taking advantage of! In this way, exercise promotes fat loss and can preferentially target visceral fat.

Exercise positively influences GLP-1 levels and function. Physical activity has been shown to increase the secretion of GLP-1, incorporating regular exercise should be a requirement of therapy with semaglutide as it can amplify the medication's benefits and is a keystone piece in transitioning to a GLP-1 lifestyle.

To maximize the benefits of exercise for gut health, metabolic optimization, and GLP-1 function, aim for approximately 150 minutes of movement a week. For any chance of sustainability, choose activities which you actually enjoy, while at the same time realizing that a well rounded exercise approach is of utmost importance. Choose a mix of low intensity movements (walking), moderate intensity movements (swimming), resistance training (weight lifting) and a fun hobby sport to tie it all together (weekend soccer) to expose yourself to the most potential benefits.

Water is essential to life, and the quality of water we consume can have significant impacts on our overall health, gut health, metabolic optimization, and the effectiveness of semaglutide. Water quality directly affects gut health, as it is involved in every digestive process. Chlorine and fluoride, commonly found in tap water, can disrupt the delicate balance of the gut microbiome. Chlorine, while effective at killing harmful pathogens, can also kill beneficial bacteria in the gut. Similarly, fluoride can have adverse effects on gut bacteria and is a too often ignored constituent of most people's drinking water. Consuming water free from these chemicals can help maintain a healthy microbiome, promoting better digestion and nutrient absorption.

The microbiome thrives in a balanced environment. High-quality water that is free from chlorine and fluoride supports the growth of beneficial bacteria and prevents dysbiosis. Furthermore, mineral-rich water provides essential nutrients that support microbial health. Minerals such as magnesium, calcium, and potassium are not only vital for human health but also for the well-being of the microbiome. These minerals can enhance microbial diversity and function, contributing to overall gut health. Hydration is crucial for metabolic processes, including energy production, nutrient transport, and waste elimination. Water that is free from contaminants supports these processes more effectively. Dehydration can impair metabolic function, leading to issues such as insulin resistance and poor glucose metabolism. Conversely, well-mineralized water supports cellular function and metabolism. Minerals like magnesium play a role in glucose regulation and insulin sensitivity, directly influencing metabolic health.

Proper hydration supports the body's natural rhythms, including circadian rhythms, which are essential for maintaining metabolic homeostasis. Adequate water intake helps regulate body temperature, hormone production, and sleep patterns. These factors are crucial for optimizing the body's GLP-1 response, as hydration can influence appetite regulation, digestion, and energy balance. Drinking quality water throughout the day helps maintain these rhythms, supporting overall health and well-being. High-quality water can enhance the effectiveness of GLP-1 receptor agonists by supporting overall metabolic health. Proper hydration ensures that the body's cells are functioning optimally, enhancing the medication's impact on appetite suppression, glucose regulation, and gastric emptying. Additionally, minerals found in quality water can support the enzymatic functions involved in these processes, making GLP-1 receptor agonists more effective.

To ensure the water you consume is of high quality, consider using water filtration systems that remove chlorine, fluoride, and other contaminants while retaining essential minerals. Reverse osmosis systems with remineralization filters are a great choice for home. Additionally, spring water is a good alternative, provided it is sourced reputably. Be aware that typical water filters for home use such as Brita do not remove fluoride from your water. You must very specifically purchase a filter with this capability, such as a Berkey filter with fluoride attachments. Aim to drink, in ounces, approximately half your weight in pounds. For a 200 pound person, you would aim to drink 100 ounces per day.

Avoiding pesticides in food is an important step toward optimizing overall health, gut health, metabolic function, and the effectiveness of semaglutide. Pesticides used in conventional farming have been demonstrated to have disastrous effects on gut health. These chemicals are designed to kill pests, but they also kill the beneficial bacteria in our gut microbiome. Consuming foods contaminated with pesticides will disrupt the delicate balance of the microbiome, leading to dysbiosis, an imbalance of gut bacteria. Studies have shown that exposure to certain pesticides can decrease the populations of Bifidobacterium and Lactobacillus species, which we already know are crucial for maintaining gut health. Pesticides can interfere with endocrine function, disrupting hormone balance and metabolic processes. Certain pesticides have been linked to insulin resistance, impairing the body's ability to regulate blood sugar levels, leading to elevated glucose levels and increased fat storage. Pesticides can interfere with the body's natural GLP-1 production and signaling pathways. These chemicals can disrupt the gut-brain axis, impairing the communication between the gut and the brain that regulates hunger and satiety.

Avoid pesticides by purchasing organic food, growing your own food or being intimately familiar with your local growing environment and the farmers within it. If you are concerned about the price of organic food, a great place to start is with organic wheat, corn and soy, as well as strictly following the "dirty dozen", which is a list of the most highly pesticide laden produce items.

Artificial flavors, colors, and preservatives can have a detrimental effect on health. These synthetic substances are not recognized by the body as natural food components, which can lead to an adverse reaction in the gut. Consuming foods with artificial additives can also disrupt the delicate balance of the microbiome. Studies have shown that certain artificial colors and preservatives can reduce the populations of important gut bacteria like those commensal species that we speak of so frequently and highly.

Artificial additives can interfere with normal metabolic processes and hormone function. For example, some artificial preservatives have been linked to endocrine disruption, which can lead to hormonal imbalances and metabolic disorders. Artificial flavors and colors can also impact appetite regulation and energy metabolism, potentially leading to overeating and weight gain. These chemicals also disrupt the gut-brain axis.

To minimize exposure to artificial flavors, colors, and preservatives, consider adopting a few potentially new practices. First, you must read every single label of any food you plan to purchase. Look for terms like artificial flavor, FD&C, and specific preservatives like sodium benzoate, potassium sorbate, TBHQ and the like. The name will sound unappetizing, this is one way to begin to learn harmful additives! Prioritize whole, unprocessed foods and packaged food with very few ingredients. Preparing meals at home allows you to control the ingredients and avoid artificial additives, which are unbelievably common in the vast majority of restaurants. Organic foods are not allowed to contain the nastiest of the artificial additives, therefore, some convenience can be had by simply buying organic.

In weaving together our environmental health, we have uncovered the profound impact that our surroundings have on our overall well-being. From the essential rays of the sun that nourish our bodies and spirits, to the purity of the water we drink, to avoidance of pesticides and artificial additives in our food to the rejuvenating power of exercise, by integrating these environmental practices into our daily lives, we create a supportive foundation for optimizing GLP-1 levels and achieving lasting health. As we move forward, let us carry the knowledge that true wellness extends beyond the confines of diet and medication, embracing the broader context of our environment. This understanding empowers us to make mindful choices that harmonize with nature, ultimately leading to a healthier, more balanced, and fulfilling life.

SECTION V: WHAT'S UNIQUE ABOUT THE GLP-1 LIFESTYLE?

CHAPTER 23: THE IMMUNE-METABOLISM CONNECTION

To lay the foundation for these discussions, it's important to understand why transitioning from losing weight while taking semaglutide to adopting a long-term GLP-1 lifestyle is so critical. This journey isn't just about the risk of gaining the weight back because you eat too much or don't exercise enough. Those habits took many decades to form, and if it were that simple, it would take many decades to reverse. The reality is more complex and boils down to a sophisticated concept known as immunometabolism. Immunometabolism is the intersection of the immune system and metabolic processes, a burgeoning field that underscores the importance of immune function in regulating metabolic health. This connection is crucial for understanding the long-term efficacy of fat loss efforts.

Throughout this book, I have alluded to the fact that our bodies are not fond of losing a significant amount of weight. Fat loss represents a stripping away of an organ-like system, a depletion of valuable future resources, and an injury to the body's metabolic balance. Like any injury, the immune system steps in to mitigate potential future losses and ensure that resources are re-sequestered. Simply put, the immune system halts further weight loss, promotes weight regain, and ideally prepares the body to store even more fat than before. Additionally, it puts mechanisms in place that make it more challenging for a similar fat loss event to occur in the future.

A very important concept in sustainable weight loss and the post-weight loss period is what I'll refer to as "offsetting." This involves ensuring that the body feels safe and content frequently throughout the weight loss process and afterward. Of course, there are many days where you will need to buckle down by eating very strictly, fasting, exercising heavily, or any combination of these. However, what most people fail to recognize is the necessity of a "safety stop" day. On these days, you reassure your body that you are not in a state of deprivation, not trying to lose every shred of fat to the point of organ failure. This may sound dramatic, but consider it in the context of human history: we are very privileged today, and this time period is but a blip in our 300,000-year history. For 99.97% of that time, we faced food insecurity and were more concerned with starvation than obesity. By demonstrating food security to the body at specific intervals during the week, we can turn off survival mechanisms and allow the body to recalibrate to the new, thinner you.

At the heart of these mechanisms lies inflammation. Imagine again that fire smoldering within your body, diverting resources away from weight loss, healthy metabolism, and organ function, creating a hostile environment for them all. My friend Joel Greene, author of "The Immunity Code," has been advocating the connection between immunity and metabolism for years, referring to it as "immune-centric fat loss." Joel's notion is that fat loss can never be sustainable in an environment where it continues to be treated like a disaster zone, full of inflammatory mediators and the body's emergency personnel. Obesity is nearly synonymous with a chronic inflammatory state, and once fat loss has occurred, it amplifies this state, making the inflammation of fat loss particularly insidious. Insulin sensitivity becomes further impaired, the remaining adipocytes function even more disrupted, metabolism slows, and hormonal imbalances take greater hold, increasing the production of cortisol and throwing leptin and ghrelin totally off track. This inflammatory response creates a cycle of metabolic dysfunction, making sustainable weight loss an oxymoron. The gut microbiome also plays a crucial role in immunometabolism, as dysbiosis can further trigger inflammation and disrupt metabolic processes, steering immunometabolism in the wrong direction.

The immune system's involvement in fat metabolism extends to the cellular level, where immune cells such as macrophages infiltrate adipose tissue and influence its function. In a healthy state, immune cells in adipose tissue help maintain homeostasis and support fat mobilization. However, in obesity, the balance shifts towards a pro-inflammatory profile, exacerbating metabolic dysfunction and hindering effective fat loss. Research supports this, showing that reducing inflammation through lifestyle interventions promotes more sustainable weight loss through immunomodulation. Macrophages play a pivotal role in regulating inflammation and fat metabolism. In conditions of chronic inflammation, often seen in obesity, macrophages shift towards an "M1" state. These M1 macrophages are characterized by pro-inflammatory properties and a tendency to promote fat storage. They act like hoarders, accumulating fat and contributing to the expansion of adipose tissue. This shift towards an M1 phenotype is driven by various factors, including excess calorie intake, a high-fat diet, and chronic inflammation.

In contrast, lean individuals typically have macrophages in an "M2" state. M2 macrophages possess anti-inflammatory properties and promote the breakdown of fat for energy. This state is conducive to metabolic health, supporting efficient fat utilization and overall homeostasis. The balance between M1 and M2 macrophages is crucial for metabolic health and is influenced by many specifics we will discuss later in this section. Interestingly, semaglutide appears to influence this macrophage balance, tipping the scales towards a more favorable M2 phenotype.

The implications of this immune-centric approach to fat loss are profound. It suggests that by supporting immune function and reducing inflammation, we can enhance the effectiveness of semaglutide and other weight loss interventions. This holistic strategy makes it more feasible to maintain weight loss, addressing the common struggle most people face after losing weight. Fortunately, semaglutide appears to alleviate many concerns regarding immunometabolism, showing reductions in dysbiosis and inflammation while positively influencing the immune system and macrophage populations. The GLP-1 lifestyle would achieve these same benefits, further supporting long-term metabolic health.

Gut health is a cornerstone of offsetting. A diet rich in specific polyphenols, prebiotics, and probiotics, timed appropriately, will foster a microbiome that can balance the immune system toward continued fat loss. We need to integrate foods known for their anti-inflammatory properties, such as omega-3 fatty acids found in fish and the polyphenol-rich fruits and vegetables. By reducing inflammation, these foods support overall metabolic health and enhance the body's ability to lose fat.

Polyphenol-rich foods are at the forefront of re-building the gut and offsetting the injury of fat loss due to their powerful anti-inflammatory properties and ability to preferentially potentiate beneficial species of bacteria. Berries are chock full of polyphenols and other antioxidants, while being low in sugar.

Blueberries, strawberries, blackberries and raspberries are all perfect for combating oxidative stress and inflammation. Offsetting should include regular consumption of these fruits at specific time intervals to enhance all of their tremendous benefits. We will elaborate these strategies in the next section of the book.

Green tea, known for its catechins, particularly epigallocatechin gallate (EGCG), reduces inflammation and supports fat metabolism. An offsetting program should include green tea, whether via capsules, steeped tea or matcha. Green tea can boost thermogenesis and fat oxidation, while also including antioxidant compounds that contribute to offsetting the injury of fat loss.

Omega-3 fatty acids are vital for their anti-inflammatory effects in an offsetting period. Fatty fish, such as salmon, mackerel, and sardines, are excellent sources of omega-3s, improving insulin sensitivity, reducing systemic inflammation, and supporting cardiovascular health. Additionally, flaxseeds and chia seeds, plant-based sources of omega-3s, can be easily incorporated into smoothies, salads, or yogurt. These do not offer the same bioavailability of fish or algal omega-3, in fact they provide alpha-linolenic acid (ALA) which must be converted into EPA and DHA (omega 3s). Still, they offer their own set of specific benefits, such as multiple beneficial plant compounds, fiber and minerals.

Prebiotic foods play a crucial role in offsetting and rebuilding the gut. Inulin supports the growth of these beneficial bacteria and enhances gut health by improving the microbiome's diversity and function, a benefit shared by many other prebiotics. Cooked and cooled rice and potatoes are among my favorite forms of prebiotic. Not only are they enjoyable to eat, but they also deliver many grams of resistant starch. Additionally, small amounts of potato starch, acacia fiber, or green banana flour are potent sources of prebiotic starches. By small amount, I mean it. For those unfamiliar with resistant starch in the diet, start by supplementing a quarter teaspoon and only increasing every subsequent week or so.

Probiotic foods are also essential for offsetting and rebuilding the gut. Fermented foods such as sauerkraut, kimchi, kefir, and yogurt contain live cultures that help balance the gut microbiome. Studies have shown fascinating outcomes from the consumption of probiotics, including reduced levels of bloating, more regular bowel movements, reduction in small intestinal bacterial overgrowth (SIBO), and increased nutrient absorption, among many others. Even the lactic acid contained in probiotics cultured with Lactobacillus spp. offers its own set of unique, gut-balancing health effects. Plan to include probiotics in your diet every day, ideally with every meal.

There are very specific protocols in place for the timing of nutrient delivery as it pertains to offsetting the fat loss injury, rebuilding the gut, and promoting overall health. It will prove most useful for you to see this structure now, with an example week of ideal food choices. My plan is for you to see the structure of offsetting now, while reading the strategies for GLP-1 optimization in the next section. Get your favorite note taking method ready.

By carefully timing nutrient intake and focusing on specific foods throughout the day, this approach aims to optimize metabolic and immune responses, reduce systemic inflammation, and support a healthy gut microbiome—helping you keep the weight off forever. This aligns closely with the "2 day core" eating pattern approach that Joel Greene created and endorses in his book, "The Immunity Code." I have spent two decades learning and testing various eating patterns, experimenting with every new trend that has had its 15 minutes of fame. The science and practicality behind the 2 day core is extremely powerful. I use this structure every week to eat very healthy foods, at specific time intervals, while utilizing many strategies for health span, including protein-rich breakfasts, plant-based foods, and fasting. You will be able to maintain this basic pattern quite easily throughout your life.

What will happen during this week is a significant proliferation of beneficial bacteria, increasing Akkermansia, Bifidobacteria, and Lactobacillus. Naturally, there is a balancing of the gut microbiome and the multitude of benefits this provides. At the same time, we will spend days completely focused on fasting and anti-inflammatory efforts that round out the health benefits. This plan is structured to meticulously time nutrient intake, focusing on the interplay of various foods and their effects on the body. Each meal is curated for specific roles in enhancing metabolic pathways and supporting gut health. By following this protocol, you will be creating an environment that fosters sustainable weight loss and overall health.

On Monday, day 1 of our pattern, our target for the day will be the mass proliferation of beneficial bacteria. Begin your day with a substantial serving of phenol-rich berries. Choose whatever is fresh, organic, and ideally seasonal at your grocery store—my favorites are blueberries and blackberries. When I say substantial serving, aim for half a standard dinner plate full of fruit. This will load the gut with phenols and fiber. Alongside this, include a handful of nuts for a small fat bolus and additional beneficial plant compounds. Walnuts are the ideal choice due to their ability to increase adiponectin. Adiponectin, often referred to as the "skinny hormone," is found at higher levels in thin, healthy individuals. The key is to wait over three hours before eating again to allow the phytochemicals to fulfill their role in the proliferation of beneficial bacteria.

Approximately 30 minutes before your next meal, have a small preload of macadamia nuts. These nuts are rich in monounsaturated fats and mimic fasting, allowing for a fat-burning state. This is known as a "preload"[3] snack, a crucial piece of the puzzle in this eating pattern. Preloads before a meal set the stage for your digestion before a large intake of calories. These snacks, usually high in fat and/or protein, help sensitize insulin, prepare digestive enzymes, and slightly curb your appetite. By incorporating this step, you will eat less, reduce your postprandial blood glucose levels, and kickstart metabolism.

For lunch, focus on resistant starch. After spending the entire morning nurturing beneficial bacteria in your gut, it's time to feed them. Resistant starch will pass through your stomach and small intestine largely undigested, making it available for your microbiome to consume. A burrito bowl is a delicious and satisfying choice for this meal. Include a cooked and cooled combination of beans and rice, your protein of choice, a little cheese and/or sour cream, and plenty of seasonal vegetables. Adding hot sauce and/or salsa not only enhances the flavor but also provides digestive benefits from vinegar and boosts thermogenic activity from hot peppers.

---

[3] Preloads are an incredible strategy to use before going out to eat or socialize with food around!

Resistant starches serve as the perfect fuel for the postbiotic production of those all important short-chain fatty acids (SCFAs) like butyrate. Wait three hours after this meal to allow this production to occur seamlessly. About an hour before dinner, consume half an avocado or a whey protein shake with olive oil. Both options provide healthy fats, which stabilize blood sugar and promote satiety. Whey protein is particularly powerful as a preload meal, aiding muscle synthesis and increasing fat oxidation. For dinner, focus on cruciferous vegetables with a side of protein. An ideal meal could be your favorite small piece of lean protein paired with Brussels sprouts. This meal is low in calories, promoting fat burning throughout the night, and high in fiber and phytonutrients, supporting liver detoxification and enhancing digestion. This combination optimally supports the growth of beneficial bacteria cultivated throughout the day and sets the stage for amplification tomorrow.

Beginning on Tuesday, day two, remember that you spent all of yesterday cultivating beneficial bacteria. You will use their presence and production of postbiotics to amplify the results of day 2. This day is designed to enhance the metabolic and anti-inflammatory benefits of fasting while strategically incorporating nutrient-dense foods. This approach supports fat loss and promotes overall health through careful timing and selection of dietary components. Studies have shown that high levels of beneficial bacteria and the postbiotics they produce, such as butyrate, increase the effectiveness of fasting. The efforts you made yesterday are amplifying the benefits you reap today.

The fast is quite simple: you won't eat until noon. However, you'll take specific supplements to enhance the benefits of the fast. Fasting in the morning promotes autophagy, the body's natural process of removing damaged cells and regenerating new ones. This cellular cleanup supports overall health and longevity. Additionally, fasting gives your digestive system a break, allowing for normal cell turnover and reallocating resources normally used for digestion to other processes. This morning, you'll take 3 grams of a high-quality omega-3 supplement. These will amplify the cellular cleanup processes and improve metabolic health while you fast.

After noon, it's ideal to incorporate about four small, fat-rich snacks. The goal is to consume low-carbohydrate, higher-fat snacks leading up to dinner to keep you in a healing, fat-burning mode throughout the day. These snacks should be rich in omega-3 or monounsaturated fats, providing sustained energy and supporting a healthy inflammatory response. Think of options like string cheese, walnuts, macadamia nuts, avocado, chia pudding, olives or olive oil, whey shakes or fish.

End your day with a large, nutrient-dense dinner rich in protein, fat and low in carbohydrates. This approach maintains your fat-burning state throughout the night. If this seems similar to ketogenic eating, you're right. The difference is that we mix ketogenic-style days with high fruit, high carbohydrate days. The transformative power lies in this variety and specific planning. For your day 2 dinner, a meal like salmon with quinoa, cauliflower, or mixed greens would be excellent. Don't hesitate to make these meals exciting. Add vegetables, spices, healthy fats, vinegars, and hot sauces to enhance the meal's flavor and nutritional power.

A plan like this offers a lot of flexibility. You can repeat the two-day cycle as often as you like, or mix it up. As long as you adhere to the basic rules of the GLP-1 lifestyle, you can't go wrong. I will provide specific strategies to close out your week, but understand that you don't have to follow these exactly. The two-day pattern we just outlined is called the "anchor." Get this right every single week, and you'll make significant strides in your metabolic health. Proliferating beneficial bacteria one day and leveraging their fasting-amplifying powers the next creates a potent 1-2 punch for health and sustainable fat loss.

Wednesday, day 3, introduces new concepts. First thing in the morning, I want you to eat with the intention of resetting your leptin function by tailoring your eating pattern to balance hunger hormones towards satiety and optimal energy expenditure. One of the most effective ways to do this is by having a large breakfast, very high in protein. You will consume the bulk of your day's calories at breakfast, while including resistant starches, good fats and approximately 50 grams of protein.

Achieving this high-protein breakfast can be challenging. Personally, I often have four fried eggs (cooked in butter), cooled potatoes, and a whey protein shake. Drink the protein shake while cooking to benefit from the power of the preload. After this enjoyable but filling breakfast, we will fast until dinner. For dinner, we'll have a meal replacement shake, consisting of whey protein, honey, olive oil, cinnamon, yogurt, acacia fiber or another resistant starch, milk, and ice. Play with the ingredients to find a combination you find delicious. This day has specific goals: preventing weight regain, driving metabolic activity high, and lowering cortisol.

Thursday, day 4, depends on how your body is feeling. Ideally, you'll repeat day 2 (Tuesday), but if you're feeling depleted and hungry, repeat Monday instead. Remember to vary your food choices and keep it fun. This basic structure is how you should plan to eat for the rest of your life. It must be sustainable and full of foods that make you happy. I know what you're thinking, adjusting to a healthier way of eating might not make you happy, at first. Often, it's the harmful bacteria in your gut that make you crave cookies, bread, and Starbucks Frappuccinos. As you foster beneficial bacteria, you'll begin to enjoy a much broader and healthier array of produce, legumes, whole grains, and other health-promoting choices. Sounds almost too good to be true, but I assure you it is the case and backed by scientific evidence.

Friday, day 5, I like to call the "digestive day". It is very similar to day 2, however, we are specifically adding compounds that aid the digestive fire. I would suggest taking bitters and digestive enzymes with your morning water and focusing on smaller portions and light, easy to digest meals like shakes and soups throughout the day. It is up to you how much you want to eat, though I suggest it be hypocaloric (lower in calories than usual) leading into the weekend[4]. Be sure to add vinegars, bitters and hot sauces liberally to your meals and fluids; consider pineapple, papaya or their subsequent supplement forms. If you have never tried a day completely focused on ease of digestion, I think you will find it a wonderful addition to your week, as you are going to feel energetic and light.

The weekend is an opportunity to reset and prepare your body for the upcoming week while still adhering to the principles of the GLP-1 lifestyle. This time acts as a mandatory safety stop, shifting

---

[4] Speaking to calorie strategies is beyond the scope of this book, however, day 1 is meant to be eucaloric (meaning eating your baseline calorie level), day 2 is meant to be moderately hypocaloric (eating in a calorie deficit according to your baseline) and the weekend is meant to be mildly hypercaloric (eating in a calorie surplus).

the focus from fat loss to offsetting. This recalibration prepares your body for sustainable, long-term fat loss or further fat loss. Do not skip this step! One key element to incorporate is a leptin reset plus highly satiating foods and a mild calorie surplus.

On one day during the weekend, repeat the massive, healthy, high-protein breakfast from Wednesday. This breakfast should provide the bulk of your calories for the day, helping to balance your hunger hormones towards satiety and optimal energy expenditure and quell any signals of distress from your body. Try not to snack much today, but if you do, opt for the small, low-carb snacks from Day 2. For dinner, listen to your body. If you're feeling very hungry and deprived, choose a satisfying but not overly large meal, like a small grilled cheese sandwich with tomato soup. If you're not feeling deprived, have the meal replacement shake. Remember you can always lean on your calorie count as a guide.

The leptin reset breakfast can be repeated over multiple days, provided you manage the rest of the day appropriately. As long as this massive breakfast contains the bulk of your calories for the day, it's beneficial. Often, I will have a very large breakfast on both Saturday and Sunday. Just remember to try fasting until dinner and then opt for a lighter meal. This approach can be flexible, especially as you become more skilled in offsetting and understand how it applies to you for sustainable fat loss.

We have explored the principles of the GLP-1 lifestyle and how to effectively incorporate the practice of offsetting, alongside resetting hunger hormones, into a weekly routine that becomes the structure of your overarching eating pattern. It is important to note that we will not be delving much into calorie counting, deficits, or specific weight loss strategies. While these aspects are crucial for understanding the complete picture of metabolic health and fat loss, they are beyond the scope of this book. Keep in mind, you should absolutely have an idea of your basal metabolic rate (BMR) and calorie requirements according to your goals.

Our focus here is on offsetting the metabolic injury that can occur with fat loss and applying these principles to the rest of the book. By following along, you are setting yourself up for success, not just in achieving your health goals, but in maintaining them for the future.

CHAPTER 24: FOOD & GLP-1 STIMULATION

In the realm of nutrition, certain foods hold the key to unlocking a cascade of metabolic benefits, including the enhanced production of GLP-1. In this chapter, we will cover a vast array of foods that you can incorporate into your eating pattern to optimize your natural production of GLP-1 or assist semaglutide and the transition off of semaglutide.

Among these foods, fiber stands out. Insoluble fiber, which is generally non-fermentable fiber, such as cellulose found in whole grains, vegetables, and nuts, resists fermentation and passes through the gut largely unchanged. While insoluble fiber doesn't directly stimulate GLP-1 production, it plays a crucial role in maintaining a healthy gut environment. This type of fiber acts like scaffolding that supports the gut's structure and function. By providing physical bulk, it helps to maintain the integrity of the intestinal walls and supports peristalsis. This not only aids in the regular elimination of waste but also helps prevent issues such as diverticulosis and hemorrhoids. This supports the entire digestive system, providing a stable foundation for the fermentation processes, while also ensuring nutrient delivery, regular digestion, and amplification of the metabolic and appetite-regulating benefits of GLP-1.

Fermentable fiber, mostly in the form of soluble fiber, is particularly prized by the gut microbiome. In the colon, this fiber undergoes fermentation by the gut microbiota. Soluble fibers, generally speaking, are prebiotics. Fermentable fibers are the gourmet feast your gut bacteria dream about and providing them in the diet is crucial, as we discussed at length previously.

Resistant starch (RS) is an important class of fermentable fiber. It shares properties with both soluble and insoluble fiber. The vital role it plays in feeding gut bacteria cannot be understated. It is estimated that early humans consumed approximately 50 grams of RS every single day, which was instrumental in building the optimal human gut, which led to the development of the complicated gut-brain axis and human life as we know it. RS is very interesting as it is often formed after cooking and is found in most cooked and cooled grains and legumes, particularly rice, potatoes and oats. I have always found this curious and have wondered if cooking and RS played a part in the rapid development of human intelligence. Maybe we can touch on that in a future book!

Inulin, another prebiotic fiber found in foods like onions, garlic, artichokes and Jerusalem artichokes, is a favorite among Bifidobacteria, a genus of bacteria you already know to enhance GLP-1 secretion. The presence of inulin in the diet supports a thriving population of Bifidobacteria in the gut microbiome. As these bacteria proliferate, they enhance the overall fermentation process, leading to increased production of SCFAs, which then interact with the L cells in the colon, triggering a cascade of positive health promoting events in the gut. Garlic and onions, pungent alliums and staples of culinary traditions worldwide, are not just flavor enhancers; they are prebiotic powerhouses. Their unique blend of inulin and fructooligosaccharides (FOS) makes them particularly effective at nourishing beneficial bacteria in the gut.

Barley and oats, grains reminiscent of ancient harvests and rustic kitchens, are not just sources of comfort and warmth; they are nutritional powerhouses. These grains are rich in beta-glucans, a type of soluble fiber that forms a viscous gel in the gut. This gel slows down digestion, fostering a lasting sense of fullness, and acts as a prebiotic. As these microbes ferment the beta-glucans, they also release SCFAs along with other beneficial postbiotics.

Legumes, including lentils, chickpeas, black beans, and their diverse family members, are nutritional powerhouses. These foods are rich in protein, fiber, and resistant starch, and a lot of it at that! Legumes and beans are, in my opinion, the easiest way to incorporate a heap of health promoting fiber into the diet. These versatile ingredients can be easily adapted into a variety of dishes, making them a valuable addition to any healthy diet, promoting enhanced GLP-1 production, improved gut health, and better metabolic function.

By embracing a fiber-rich diet, you're not just nourishing your body; you're cultivating a thriving ecosystem within your gut. This community of microbes works tirelessly to support your health and well-being and is the cornerstone of the GLP-1 lifestyle. You will learn how to incorporate fiber successfully into your diet in the next section. However, fiber is just one part of the story.

Fatty fish, such as salmon and mackerel, are rich in omega-3 fatty acids, high-quality protein, and essential nutrients, making them a powerhouse for metabolic health. Omega-3 fatty acids are renowned for their anti-inflammatory properties, which not only support cardiovascular health but also aid in maintaining a healthy gut environment. The high protein content in fatty fish promotes satiety, helping individuals feel full longer and thereby reducing overall caloric intake. Research has demonstrated that consuming fatty fish can enhance GLP-1 secretion. Given these multifaceted benefits, incorporating fatty fish into one's diet is a vital component of the GLP-1 lifestyle.

Dairy products, such as milk, cheese, and yogurt, independently contribute to weight loss and offer benefits for maintaining weight loss. Dairy promotes satiety, reduces overall caloric intake by controlling hunger and has been shown in studies to independently support the production of GLP-1. The nutrient density and protein content in dairy helps to control appetite. Dairy has been demonstrated, study after study, to aid in weight loss, metabolic health, muscle gain and to reduce weight re-gain.

Fermented dairy products take the effects of dairy and take it up a notch. Products like yogurt and kefir contain probiotics, lactic acid and metabolites that all balance gut health and turn the tide on metabolic health, GLP-1 production, and sustainable weight management. Fermented dairy is one of the superfoods that make the GLP-1 lifestyle so powerful. Greek yogurt, a protein-dense dairy product, offers multiple health benefits. It contains all benefits of fermented dairy while also contributing very high levels of protein, which regulates appetite, making it a valuable addition to any weight management plan. Studies have even shown that incorporating yogurt can contribute to weight loss and assist in preventing weight regain.

Whey protein, derived from milk, stands out as a complete protein source containing all essential amino acids and is known for its high bioavailability and rapid absorption. Studies have shown that whey protein significantly increases GLP-1 levels. Additionally, whey protein is top tier for support of muscle repair and growth. Given its ease of use and versatility, whey protein is a must have in the GLP-1 lifestyle pantry.

Legumes, including beans and lentils, are another valuable protein source, outside of their value for fiber content. Hopefully you are beginning to realize why the healthiest societies in the world eat a lot of legumes. They are a true superfood, much more real in this sense than fads like açai berry (açai has its benefits, but calling it a superfood is a stretch). They are rich in plant-based protein, fiber, and complex carbohydrates, with a low glycemic index that ensures a gradual release of glucose into the bloodstream. This combination makes them highly satiating and health promoting.

Incorporating a variety of protein sources, including fatty fish, whey protein, fermented dairy and legumes into the diet can significantly enhance GLP-1 production and support weight management. These foods not only contribute to effective weight loss but also help prevent weight regain. Understanding and utilizing protein provides an important piece of a comprehensive approach to optimizing GLP-1 levels.

Fats play a significant role, as well. Incorporating sources of healthy fats such as avocados, coconut oil and butter can enhance the benefits of semaglutide and are considered crucial to the GLP-1 lifestyle.

Monounsaturated fats, which are well-documented for their cardio-protective properties, help reduce levels of low-density lipoprotein (LDL) cholesterol, which, in the setting of inflammation and oxidation, is the cholesterol that is concerning for cardiovascular disease. Monounsaturated fats can actually increase HDL, or "good" cholesterol, completely flipping your cholesterol ratio toward heart health. This ratio is important for reducing the risk of cardiovascular diseases, including heart attacks and strokes. Foods rich in monounsaturated fats include olive oil and macadamia nuts, stalwart dietary contributors of overall health.

Monounsaturated fats are particularly rich in compounds like oleic acid, which possess anti-inflammatory properties that help reduce chronic inflammation in the body, which you now know to be rather detrimental to overall health. They also play a significant role in improving insulin sensitivity and blood sugar control. Additionally, monounsaturated fats can positively impact GLP-1 levels, enhancing their production and secretion. They often come packaged with other beneficial nutrients that further support metabolic health. For instance, olive oil contains plant compound antioxidants like polyphenols, which work synergistically with monounsaturated fats to reduce oxidative stress and inflammation. These combined effects can enhance overall health and optimize metabolic processes, including the regulation of GLP-1 levels.

Olive oil, particularly speaking to extra virgin olive oil (EVOO), is rich in monounsaturated fats and antioxidants. It deserves its reputation as a longtime staple of a healthy diet. It has been shown to have numerous health benefits, including reducing inflammation, improving heart health, and supporting a healthy gut. Olive oil's healthy fat content can enhance GLP-1 production and liberally drizzling this oil on salads, vegetables, and other dishes can improve the nutrient profile of meals and support a GLP-1 lifestyle.

Avocados are special. They contain heaps of super healthy plant fat but are also a good source of fiber. This combination of healthy fats and fiber is very unique and makes avocado another true superfood contender, especially given that they also have a high nutrient density, with significant levels of vitamins E, K, and B, along with potassium.

Coconut oil is a pretty amazing fat source and is quite beneficial, due to its unique inclusion of medium-chain triglycerides (MCTs) and saturated fats like lauric acid. Lauric acid is a type of saturated fat with potent antimicrobial properties, which helps to maintain a healthy gut environment by combating harmful bacteria, viruses, and fungi. Research has shown that MCTs can enhance the secretion of GLP-1 and that coconut oil in the diet can also aid in weight management independently by promoting satiety and improving fat metabolism. The MCTs in coconut oil are metabolized differently than other fats; they are transported directly to the liver, where they are rapidly converted into ketones. Ketones are an alternative energy source for the body, particularly the brain, and can help reduce hunger and support mental clarity.

Furthermore, the regular use of coconut oil in cooking or as a dietary supplement can contribute to better overall fat metabolism. This can lead to improved energy expenditure and a greater ability to burn fat. By promoting a sense of fullness and enhancing metabolic processes, coconut oil can play a supportive role in a diet aimed at optimizing GLP-1 levels and metabolic health.

Butter, always of the high-quality grass-fed variety, offers a rich source of healthy saturated fats, conjugated linoleic acid (CLA), and essential fat-soluble vitamins such as A, D, E, and K2. Grass-fed butter is distinct from conventional butter due to its higher nutritional content, derived from cows that graze on pasture rather than being fed a grain-based diet. You should get used to purchasing food from animals that are happy, the effect on our bodies is great.

Grass-fed butter is an excellent source of healthy saturated fats. These fats are crucial for maintaining cellular integrity, as they form the structure of cell membranes, ensuring proper cell function and resilience. Saturated fats also play a vital role in hormone production, ones like GLP-1. CLA has been extensively studied for its health benefits, particularly in the context of metabolic health and fat loss. Research suggests that CLA can improve body composition by reducing body fat and increasing lean muscle mass. It is also associated with enhanced insulin sensitivity and reduced inflammation. Fat soluble vitamins play various critical roles in maintaining health and most are deficient in the modern diet. To quickly summarize, Vitamin A is essential for vision, immune function, and skin health. Vitamin D supports nearly everything, but is most well known for bone health, immune function and mood regulation. Vitamin E acts as a powerful antioxidant, protecting cells from oxidative damage and supporting skin and immune health. We touched on vitamin K2 already, you hopefully recall its importance in bone health and cardiovascular health by its shuttling of calcium to appropriate areas of the body.

Saturated fats in coconut oil and butter help support the production of GLP-1, and the presence of CLA in butter further supports fat loss and improves body composition, making these fats a valuable addition to the GLP-1 lifestyle. Hooray for your taste buds!

Nuts and seeds, such as almonds, walnuts, chia seeds, and flaxseeds, support GLP-1 production independently by promoting a healthy gut microbiome and through anti-inflammatory properties that benefit overall metabolic health. I suggest limiting nuts and most seeds as the calorie content to nutrient ratio typically does not make them a useful addition to most people's eating pattern. In fact, it can be disastrous for weight loss goals. One tiny tbsp of peanut butter is 100 calories, and I bet you can't stop at one. Additionally, the fats are mostly omega 6, which you don't need more of in your diet. All in all, skip any nut and seed butters and eat whole nuts and seeds very sparingly. My favorites are walnuts and macadamia nuts. I already spoke earlier about these two; walnuts containing adiponectin and macadamia nuts monounsaturated fats.

Now, an exception are the tiny titans of nutrition, chia and flax seeds. These are packed with soluble fiber, beneficial fatty acids, and lignans, compounds with potent anti-inflammatory and antioxidant properties. Chia and flax seeds provide a multitude of health benefits and a subtle yet impactful GLP-1 boost. I would not avoid these seeds as they rank high on the nutrient density: calorie ratio.

Grapefruit is a potent activator of adenosine monophosphate-activated protein kinase (AMPK), an enzyme crucial for maintaining cellular energy balance. AMPK acts as a metabolic master switch, promoting fat burning by increasing the body's ability to oxidize fatty acids. It also regulates energy production and consumption within the body. Interestingly, AMPK and GLP-1 mutually enhance each other, making grapefruit particularly effective at curbing appetite and promoting fat burning. For example, you can amplify the fasting state by having three or four grapefruits alone for breakfast on day two. Don't hesitate to incorporate this powerful fruit into your routine for its remarkable metabolic benefits.

Next, let's talk about dark berries. I've already shared my enthusiasm for berries, but it's worth emphasizing their incredible health benefits once more. Dark-hued berries are the cream of the crop when it comes to healthy fruit. These nutritional powerhouses are rich in phenolic compounds, fiber, and pectin. They have the remarkable ability to rebuild your microbiome, improve cardiovascular health, and significantly enhance metabolic health. Don't hesitate to enjoy a generous portion of these berries. They are best consumed with a small amount of fat on the morning of day one and then left alone to digest for over three hours.

I am not a fan of elimination diets, with one very important exception. It's essential to improve your diet as a whole, not just by adding healthier foods but also by removing harmful ones. We've discussed how processed foods, refined flour, refined sugar, and other unhealthy ingredients disrupt metabolic health, damage your gut microbiome, and interfere with GLP-1 signaling. The first items to eliminate should be sugary, calorie-laden drinks, as they can significantly undermine your dietary efforts. It's like taking three steps forward and two steps back until you remove these "food" items from your routine.

Eliminating these sugary drinks can be challenging, especially if you're used to a morning sugar rush, often in the form of a double caramel latte or something similar. Unfortunately, this habit has to go and there aren't many easy ways to replace it. One easy drink swap can be replacing sugary sodas and artificial sweeteners with naturally flavored sparkling water, as there are many excellent brands and flavors available these days. For snacks, replace processed options with healthier alternatives like a handful of walnuts, a cheese stick, an avocado, high-quality meat or jerky, yogurt, or a protein shake. This approach will help you build a healthier, more sustainable diet and significantly improve your metabolic health.

Restaurants often use cheap, health-destroying ingredients to buy in bulk and increase profit margins. This can be difficult to avoid, but you can save a lot of money and significantly improve your health by embracing cooking at home. Cooking is a unique and wonderful skill, gifted only to humans, so enjoy the experience! Invest in cookbooks, follow Instagram chefs, and experiment with spices and herbs to create flavorful dishes that are both healthy and satisfying. With the foundational principles of the GLP-1 lifestyle, it becomes phenomenally easy to prepare nutritious meals at home.

For instance, compare the ingredients and nutrition facts of your favorite restaurant's fried rice to your homemade version. Using wild rice cooked in coconut oil, fresh organic vegetables, and wild-caught shrimp creates a dish that is an explosion of health benefits. In contrast, restaurant versions are often gut bombs filled with unhealthy fats, artificial ingredients and low-quality substitutes, forcing you to offset your next couple of meals. By making these changes, you can enjoy delicious, nutrient-rich foods that support your overall health.

Much like the interest of a well-managed retirement account accrues astonishingly over decades, the power of compounding affects our bodies similarly in terms of eating patterns. It's not necessary to make perfect decisions at every meal, but consistently choosing well and incorporating a variety of foods that support a GLP-1 lifestyle will undoubtedly begin to compound health benefits, paying dividends for the rest of your life. Each nutritious choice works synergistically with the next, driving your health upward. This positive spiral leads to changes in body composition, improved metabolic health, and enhanced mood, which further motivates you to continue making great decisions.

Look around you and it becomes clear; poor choices also compound, leading to a downward spiral where unhealthy decisions beget more unhealthy decisions. This negative cycle can severely impact your health. An intelligent, balanced approach aimed at the GLP-1 lifestyle supports weight management, metabolic health, mood, parenting, and everything else that impacts your overall quality of life. By understanding the role of these foods in the body, you can make informed choices today that set the stage for a healthier future.

CHAPTER 25: DO YOU NEED TO TAKE SUPPLEMENTS?

In the pursuit of optimal metabolic health, the role of supplements in enhancing GLP-1 production and efficacy cannot be overlooked. While exercise, diet, and lifestyle practices provide the foundation, a specific complement of supplements offer additional support for boosting GLP-1 levels and are worthy of your consideration, if your budget allows. This chapter delves into the scientific basis for using supplements to augment GLP-1 activity and explores the most effective supplements for achieving metabolic health.

Berberine is one of the most well-studied supplements for GLP-1 optimization. This plant alkaloid has been shown to enhance GLP-1 secretion and improve insulin sensitivity, making it a potent ally in the fight against metabolic disease. Berberine works by activating AMPK, which we learned about in our discussion on grapefruit. Activation of AMPK promotes GLP-1 secretion and can significantly enhance the body's natural GLP-1 production. Berberine is a plant compound found in several herbs, including goldenseal, barberry, and Oregon grape. It has been used in traditional medicine for centuries and has recently gained attention for its potential to improve metabolic health. Studies have shown that berberine supplementation can improve blood sugar control, reduce insulin resistance, and support weight loss.

One mechanism through which berberine enhances GLP-1 is by modulating gut microbiota, in which berberine has been shown to positively alter the composition of the microbiome. Furthermore, berberine has been found to inhibit dipeptidyl peptidase-4 (DPP-4), an enzyme that degrades GLP-1. By inhibiting DPP-4, berberine prolongs the action of GLP-1, enhancing its effects. This dual action—boosting GLP-1 production and inhibiting its degradation—makes berberine a particularly powerful supplement for improving metabolic health.

Clinical studies have demonstrated the benefits of berberine in various populations. For instance, a study published in the journal *Metabolism* found that berberine supplementation significantly improved glucose and lipid metabolism in patients with type 2 diabetes. Another study in the *Journal of Clinical Endocrinology & Metabolism* showed that berberine reduced insulin resistance and body weight in obese individuals.

Omega-3 fatty acids have already been discussed, but are a go to supplement for GLP-1 enhancement. The omega-3s, eicosapentaenoic acid (EPA) and docosahexaenoic acid (DHA), achieve their anti-inflammatory effects by influencing the production of cytokines and eicosanoids, which are signaling molecules involved in the inflammatory response. EPA and DHA can decrease the production of pro-inflammatory cytokines while increasing the production of anti-inflammatory ones. This shift in the inflammatory balance helps protect the gut lining and maintain the integrity of the intestinal barrier. In addition, they improve insulin sensitivity. Research supports the benefits of omega-3 fatty acids in enhancing GLP-1 activity. A study published in the *American Journal of Clinical Nutrition* found that omega-3 supplementation increased GLP-1 levels in individuals with metabolic syndrome. Another study in *Diabetes Care* demonstrated that omega-3 supplementation improved insulin sensitivity and reduced inflammation in people with type 2 diabetes. These studies highlight the potential of omega-3 fatty acids to support overall metabolic health.

Probiotics play a significant role in supporting GLP-1 production, as we have learned. The vast majority of probiotics exert a positive effect, however a few are particularly potent. Certain strains of Lactobacillus and Bifidobacterium have been shown to enhance GLP-1 secretion, such as Lactobacillus rhamnosus GG (LGG), Lactobacillus acidophilus and Bifidobacterium lactis BB-12, amongst the others we discussed previously. Single strain or species probiotic therapy is an emerging health technology and one I suggest you adopt sooner rather than later. Studies have demonstrated significant improvements in the health of the gut with specific strains and species known for enhancing gut health and supporting immune function, like the ones listed above.

Magnesium is another critical nutrient for GLP-1 optimization. Magnesium deficiency is common and can negatively impact insulin sensitivity and glucose metabolism. Magnesium is a co-factor in over 300 biochemical reactions in the body, suffice to say healthy levels of this mineral are rather important! Many of those 300 plus reactions involve proper function of the pancreas and other metabolic processes that tie closely to GLP-1 optimization. There are several forms of magnesium, each with unique benefits. Magnesium citrate is great for quick absorption and digestive health. Magnesium glycinate promotes relaxation and reduces anxiety. Magnesium malate supports energy production and muscle function, while magnesium threonate benefits cognitive function. Other beneficial forms include magnesium oxide for general use and magnesium chloride for better hydration.

Using a magnesium complex that combines these types is often the best choice for comprehensive benefits.

Curcumin, the active compound in turmeric, is renowned for its anti-inflammatory and antioxidant properties. Curcumin has been shown to enhance GLP-1 secretion by reducing inflammation and oxidative stress in the gut. To maximize curcumin's benefits, it is often combined with black pepper extract, specifically piperine, which enhances its bioavailability by inhibiting certain metabolic processes that would otherwise limit curcumin absorption. Interestingly, it is actually best if you can find a turmeric or curcumin supplement without any black pepper or piperine. You are not looking for bioavailability in this instance. We want the curcumin to stay in the gut, as any levels that are transferred to the bloodstream will not be available to work their anti-inflammatory magic within the digestive system. This is a current controversy amongst curcumin supplement manufacturers, but when you are particularly targeting the gut, the choice is clear.

In addition to these specific supplements, maintaining adequate levels of vitamin D is crucial for GLP-1 production. Sun exposure is the truest means to boost vitamin D levels, as it allows the body to produce vitamin D3 through skin exposure to UVB rays. However, if you are struggling with natural vitamin D production, supplementation may become necessary. If you must supplement with vitamin D, make the most of it. Take 5,000-10,000 IU daily for a short burst - up to a week. This approach ensures that the benefits of vitamin D on GLP-1 are fully realized, while also allowing you to transition to natural vitamin D production once chronic inflammation subsides.

Alpha-Lipoic Acid (ALA) is a naturally occurring compound essential for energy metabolism and known for its powerful antioxidant properties. It has been extensively studied for its benefits in improving glucose metabolism and insulin sensitivity, and recent research highlights its potential in enhancing GLP-1 production and function. ALA boosts GLP-1 production through protection of L-cells from oxidative damage and improved insulin sensitivity through AMPK activation. Additionally, ALA supports cellular energy metabolism by acting as a cofactor for mitochondrial enzymes involved in the Krebs cycle, ensuring that intestinal cells have the energy needed to produce and release GLP-1 efficiently. Clinical studies demonstrate that ALA supplementation can improve insulin sensitivity, reduce fasting blood glucose levels, and enhance overall metabolic health.

In addition to these core supplements, several other herbs and nutrients have been identified for their potential to enhance GLP-1 production and function. Most of these are easy to incorporate in some way, so I would suggest that you do so. These natural compounds offer a variety of mechanisms to support metabolic health.

Ginger has been shown to influence GLP-1 secretion, as it contains bioactive compounds such as gingerols and shogaols, which exhibit anti-inflammatory and antioxidant properties. Studies have demonstrated that ginger supplementation can enhance the secretion of GLP-1, reduce inflammation and oxidative stress, and create a favorable environment for GLP-1 production and action.

Cinnamon is another spice with potent metabolic benefits, containing compounds such as cinnamaldehyde, which can enhance the production of GLP-1. Regular consumption of cinnamon can improve glucose regulation and support better appetite control by enhancing GLP-1 secretion and its effects.

Fenugreek seeds are rich in soluble fiber and have been traditionally used to improve digestive health and metabolic function. Fenugreek has been shown to stimulate GLP-1 secretion, likely due to its high fiber content and its ability to modulate the gut microbiome. Additionally, fenugreek can improve insulin sensitivity and reduce blood glucose levels.

Aloe vera is known for its soothing and healing properties, but it also has significant metabolic benefits. Studies have shown that aloe vera gel can enhance the secretion of GLP-1 and improve insulin sensitivity. Aloe vera's anti-inflammatory properties help create a healthy intestinal environment conducive to GLP-1 production.

Bitter melon, a vegetable commonly used in Asian cuisine and traditional medicine, has been shown to improve glucose metabolism and enhance GLP-1 secretion. Bitter melon contains compounds such as charantin and polypeptide-p, which exhibit insulin-like effects. These compounds help improve insulin sensitivity and promote the release of GLP-1.

Quercetin is a flavonoid found in various fruits, vegetables, and herbs, including apples, onions, and capers. It has strong anti-inflammatory and antioxidant properties. Quercetin has been shown to enhance GLP-1 secretion by modulating the gut microbiome and reducing oxidative stress.

Ginseng, particularly Panax ginseng, is a well-known adaptogenic herb that has been used for centuries to enhance energy and overall health. Ginsenosides, the active compounds in ginseng, have been shown to stimulate GLP-1 secretion and improve insulin sensitivity. Ginseng's ability to reduce inflammation and support gut health further enhances its benefits for GLP-1 production and metabolic regulation.

Green tea has been shown to improve insulin sensitivity and promote the secretion of GLP-1. Regular consumption of green tea or its extracts can support metabolic health by enhancing GLP-1 production and function, aiding in appetite regulation and glucose control.

By incorporating these supplements into a comprehensive health routine that includes the entirety of the GLP-1 lifestyle; wise food choices, regular exercise and lifestyle modifications, you can effectively boost GLP-1 production and enhance its metabolic effects. The synergistic interaction between these supplements and the body's natural processes creates an optimal hormonal environment, supporting better glucose regulation, appetite control, and overall metabolic health.

Transitioning from using semaglutide for weight loss to adopting a long-term GLP-1 lifestyle is crucial for sustainable results. This process is complex and involves immunometabolism, the intersection of immune function and metabolic processes. Offsetting the injury to fat loss is foundational not only during weight loss, but also to long term maintenance. These days reassure the body that it is not in a state of deprivation, helping to turn off survival mechanisms and recalibrate to a healthier state. Reducing chronic inflammation and shifting the immune system back to health promotion is mission critical.

We have explored various foods and supplements that play a critical role in enhancing GLP-1 production and improving metabolic health. Incorporating specific foods while supplementing in a highly specific manner is cornerstone to the GLP-1 lifestyle and puts you directly on track for continued weight loss and improved metabolic health.

In the upcoming final section, we will put together highly practical advice for implementing the GLP-1 lifestyle over the course of a month. This comprehensive plan will include detailed food suggestions, supplementation guidelines and lifestyle practices designed to put you in the driver's seat of your new GLP-1 lifestyle. By following this structured approach, you can effectively harness the power of GLP-1 to achieve better metabolic health and overall well-being, while learning the tools to take over the wheel for the rest of your life.

SECTION VI: THE LIFESTYLE, SUMMARIZED

CHAPTER 26: NOW IT'S YOUR TURN

Congratulations, you've made it to the final chapter of our journey in building a GLP-1 lifestyle. This is a significant milestone, and you should be proud of your dedication and perseverance. In this chapter, we will summarize all the information you've absorbed into practical, bite-sized chunks. Alongside the notes you took throughout the book, this is the chapter to return to time and time again.

Please join my Facebook group titled "The GLP-1 Lifestyle." This group is tailored specifically to the content of this book, providing a space for you to connect with others, share experiences, ask questions, and receive additional guidance. It's a supportive community where you can find motivation and practical advice from people who are on the same journey as you.
Here's the website for easier access: https://www.facebook.com/groups/glp1lifestyle.

Also, please sign up with Fullscript for convenient and discounted means to your key supplements. First, create a Fullscript account, then sign up with my dispensary and take a look at the template "GLP-1 Lifestyle". Here you can purchase every recommended supplement with the push of a button. I only chose brands that I have personally used and can vouch for their dedication to the highest quality manufacturing. All of this and at a 25% discount for you. Here's the website: https://us.fullscript.com/welcome/drhacketthealth.

Moving on, and this is important. I want you to discuss any symptoms you are experiencing with your primary care provider as they may wish to tailor your dose accordingly. However, remember that the mild and common side effects typically diminish over time as your body adapts to the medication.

Understand the basic symptoms associated with severe side effects of semaglutide.

Symptoms of Pancreatitis

- Pain: Severe abdominal pain that often spreads to your back.
- Accompanying: Nausea and vomiting.

Symptoms of Gallbladder Issues

- Pain: Severe pain in the upper right side of the abdomen.
- Accompanying: Fever, jaundice (yellowing of the skin and eyes), or changes in stool color.

Symptoms of Kidney Injury

- Urine Output: Changes in urine output.
- Swelling: Swelling in the legs and ankles.
- Fatigue: Unusual, noteworthy fatigue.

Symptoms of Severe Allergic Reactions

- Skin: Rash, itching.
- Swelling: Swelling of the face, lips, tongue, or throat.
- Respiratory: Difficulty breathing.

Symptoms of Thyroid Tumors

- Lump: Lump or swelling in the neck.
- Swallowing: Difficulty swallowing.
- Voice: Hoarse voice.

Seek prompt care with any of these signs or symptoms.

Calorie counting is based off of your Basal Metabolic Rate (BMR) plus activity level. This is the amount of calories you burn as a function of your bodily processes, taking into account some personalized factors. Essentially, the level of calories you burn when you are going about your typical day.

To determine your BMR plus activity, I like to use the online calculator from calculator.net (Calculator.net BMR Calculator). This will give you your daily calorie burn, which we define as your 100% calorie rate. The pattern I want you to commit to memory and use from now on is as follows:

Day 1 Pattern

- Caloric Intake: 90-100% of your BMR plus activity level.
- Breakfast, wait 3 hours; lunch, wait 3 hours, dinner.
- Refer to section 5, chapter 23 for specifics on any of the daily eating patterns you are meant to utilize.

Day 2 Pattern

- Caloric Intake: 80% of your BMR plus activity level.
- Take amplified fast supplements, do not eat until noon; ok to have protein and fat rich snacks throughout the day before dinner.

Offsetting Days

- Caloric Intake: 100-110% of your BMR plus activity level.
- Very large high protein breakfast; highly enjoyable, satiating foods.
- Considered a feast day and should be utilized at least once per week

You don't need to go outside this structure. Keeping it simple ensures that you can follow the plan without getting bogged down in complex calculations or restrictive diets. By following this very simple guideline, you introduce time restriction, fasting and feasting into your lifestyle. By varying your intake in this manner, you can support your metabolic health and flexibility while maintaining a balanced approach to eating.

Eat the vast majority of your food when the sun is out (all of it during the summer), stop eating after 8 PM, every single day.

The secondary approach to eating involves the specific foods you will be incorporating to optimize your GLP-1 lifestyle.

Fatty Fish

- Examples: Salmon, halibut, any "small fish" like mackerel or sardines.
- Serving Size: Aim for 20 grams, in a tinned variety this would be approximately 1 tin.
- Cooking Methods: From the tin, grilled or baked
- Pairing: GLP-1 lifestyle approved fats, vegetables, and whole grains (see below).
- Suggested Brand: Look for brands that are wild, line caught or have healthful, sustainable farming practices; look for fresh fish from a local natural grocer for salmon and halibut, while Wild Planet is a fantastic source of tinned fish.

Fermented Dairy

- Examples: kefir, yogurt.
- Serving Size: 1-2 cups, depending on meal and calorie goals.
- Usage: Day 1 breakfast, day 2 break-fast, "massive" breakfast day, high protein snack, preload before a meal (very versatile).

- Pairing: Berries, grapefruit, chia seeds, coconut oil, olive oil, fiber supplements, whey protein.
- Suggested Brand: grass fed and organic is very important; not only are animals treated with dignity but their products contain such greater levels of micronutrients and lack inflammatory mediators found in factory farmed products.
- Note: consider making your own homemade yogurt, as I do; do it correctly from the start and buy a sous vide machine. They offer perfect temperature regulation and convenience, it's worth the upfront purchase. Mix two capsules of probiotics, 1 tablespoon of potato starch, and stir well in half a gallon of whole milk. Set the sous vide machine set to 100°F for 36 hours. This method ensures a potent dose of beneficial bacteria in a delicious form. For the second batch, use the first batch yogurt as your inoculation, this saves expensive probiotic capsules and makes a better, creamier and more consistent yogurt. Experiment with different strains of probiotics!

Butter & Coconut Oil

- Serving Size: A tbsp at a time.
- Usage: These should be your staples for cooking; coconut oil can also be added to yogurt, smoothies and salads.
- Suggested Brand: Organic or grass fed butter, organic coconut oil (for efficiency, Kerrygold butter and Kirkland brand coconut oil are priced great at Costco).

Extra Virgin Olive Oil

- Serving Size: A tbsp at a time.
- Usage: Only eat olive oil raw from now on; use it on salads, pizza, pasta, in shakes and standalone in a shot glass from time to time.

- Suggested Brand: Organic, high polyphenol, extra virgin olive oil is what you are looking for in order to take advantage of the health benefits. Paleovalley makes a very good oil if you are interested in a premium product; otherwise the organic version at Costco will suffice.

Whey Protein

- Serving Size: Approximately 20 grams.
- Usage: Pre-workout, post-workout, pre-load before a meal, part of a meal replacement shake, added to yogurt during "massive" breakfast day.
- Pairing: yogurt, berries, milk.
- Suggested Brands: Dr. Mercola Pure Power, Paleovalley, NorCal Organic.

Legumes

- Examples: Black beans, kidney beans, pinto beans, navy beans (you get the point), also lentils and chickpeas.
- Serving Size: The only limit is in regard to your personal fiber tolerance.
- Cooking Method: buy canned or pre-cooked; otherwise be sure to either soak them overnight or cook them for an extended period of time. Also, clear the water while they soak or cook and strain canned beans; this liquid contains plant compounds that can further exacerbate mild gastrointestinal distress.
- Usage: Incredibly versatile; salads, soups, Indian food, Mexican food, homemade burgers.
- Pairing: on the side of practically everything…
- Suggested Brand: go for organic; legumes are cheap and are sprayed with a lot of pesticides; Costco offers flats of black beans, kidney beans and garbanzo beans (chickpeas).

- Note: Chickpeas are particularly potent for their fat burning potential and are as versatile as a food gets.

Vegetables

- Examples: cruciferous veggies (broccoli, cauliflower, Brussels sprouts, cabbage), leafy greens (spinach, kale, arugula), green beans, peppers, winter squashes (butternut, kabocha); almost anything else, its hard to go wrong.
- Cooking Method: Steamed, sautéed, or included in salads.
- Usage: Endless and their usage is limitless; never concern yourself with eating too many vegetables.
- Pairing: Cooking them in GLP-1 lifestyle approved fats levels up the health benefits.
- Suggested Brand: Try your best to get local and also organic (often times local will not be certified organic but spray free, get to a know a local farmer).

Prebiotic Vegetables

- Examples: Garlic, onion, leeks, scapes, scallions, artichokes, Jerusalem artichokes.
- Cooking Method: Raw, sautéed with butter, caramelized or steamed (mainly, artichokes).
- Usage: Add to every meal; the starting point of a majority of gourmet home cooked meals is diced garlic and onion simmering in butter.
- Pairing: There ins't much that garlic and sautéed onions don't go with!
- Suggested Brand: Organic is not as critical here, though clearly a good practice.

Potatoes

- Examples: Russet, red, blue, yellow, sweet potato, yam.

- Serving Size: Approximately 1 russet potato sized amount.
- Usage: Potato salad, baked potatoes, breakfast potatoes, homemade steak fries, spiraled noodles (in the case of sweet potatoes), there are many delicious options.
- Cooking Method: No deep fried potatoes!
- Pairing: Cook them gently with GLP-1 lifestyle approved fats.
- Suggested Brand: Organic, these are a high pesticide crop.
- Note: Potatoes have been shown time and time again to support healthy weight and to be an important crop in healthy cultures, consume them in a GLP-1 lifestyle approved way and enjoy the delicious reward.

Whole Grains

- Examples: Quinoa, brown rice, barley, oats, farro, amaranth.
- Serving Size: about a 1/4-1/3 dinner plate sized amount.
- Cooking Method: soak and cook in a similar fashion to legumes; whole grains do extremely well being "finished" with a butter sauté.
- Usage: Serve as a side dish, base for vegetable and protein bowls or in a sautéed variety with GLP-1 lifestyle approved fats.
- Suggested Brand: Much of the controversy surrounding farming practices and pesticide use in the United States, including heavy glyphosate (Roundup) use, surround whole grains. For this reason, I strongly suggest purchasing organic and as local as possible.
- Note: Oatmeal is a wonderful, healthy choice that pairs very well with the second meal on Day 1 (3 hours after your berry meal). The great thing about oatmeal is the super satiating fiber and protein load it provides and the ability to customize it with a myriad of other GLP-1 approved food choices.

Fruit

- Examples: Dark fruits, particularly berries (blueberries, blackberries) or cherries, grapefruit.
- Serving Size: depends on usage; if it is your Day 1, you will eat a lot, about half a dinner plate's worth. If they are part of a snack, maybe 1/2 to 1 cup; if you are eating grapefruit to amplify your fast, it could be 3-4 grapefruits.
- Usage: Yogurt, shakes, standalone with a small handful of fat on Day 1, as part of a snack on Day 2, etc.
- Brand: All creatures like berries, insects included. These are heavily sprayed crops, buy organic.

Avocado

- Serving Size: 1/2 to 1 avocado.
- Usage: Anytime fat is desired as part of your day's eating plans or in the case of requiring further satiation. Add to salads, toast, shakes or on the side of anything with a little salt and pepper.
- Suggested Brand: Given their hard exterior, these are not necessary to purchase organic.

Nuts and Seeds

- Examples: Macadamia nuts, walnuts.
- Serving Size: Small handful at a time.
- Usage: As part of the large berry meal in the morning of Day 1, as a small fat snack on Day 2.
- Pairing: Eat with your berries, add to yogurt, salads or have standalone.
- Suggested Brand: visit the bulk section of your local natural grocer.

Chia Seeds

- Serving Size: A few tbsps.
- Usage: Add to yogurt, shakes or water with lemon or apple cider vinegar, or make chia pudding.
- Note: if adding to water, be sure to give it time to soak and stir frequently.

Part of the GLP-1 lifestyle is consuming large amounts of fiber, including insoluble, soluble, pectin and resistant starch. However, it is critically important that you build your tolerance to consuming higher levels of fiber. The gastrointestinal distress that can occur by going too much, too fast can be extremely uncomfortable. Not to mention, you are likely to be very unpopular in your house and may be spending some time alone!

Fortunately, I'm providing you with a step-by-step strategy and I want you to be very diligent with this. If you take it too far, you'll know later that day…

Start Very Slow

- Legumes are an easy way to test your fiber tolerance, don't worry about adding fiber supplements until your tolerance is acceptable.
- Some people have incredibly delicate digestive systems when beginning this process. It is not unheard of for five garbanzo beans to cause GI distress.
- Begin to test yourself, knowing how much fiber you consume already.
- In extreme examples, some people increase their tolerance by one garbanzo bean a week!

- If you can eat a fibrous meal like a bean burrito, chana masala, bean soup, etc; go ahead and begin experimenting with fiber supplements (see below).

Hydrate

- You will want to start drinking more water.
- Fiber has absorbent qualities and will otherwise dehydrate your digestive system.

Diversity of Source

- Naturally, this process of GLP-1 optimization will incorporate a diversity of fiber sources to your system.
- This builds your tolerance and optimizes the microbiome all its own.
- Your only job here otherwise is paying attention to what you are introducing and in what quantities, and adjusting "dose" as need be.

Prebiotic supplements are important, eventually, because obtaining appropriate levels can be difficult to achieve. I say eventually because one must have solid gut health and a lack of dysbiosis in order to avoid uncomfortable side effects while using prebiotic supplements.

Inulin

- Benefits: Powerfully feeds beneficial gut bacteria and supports metabolic health.
- Usage: Use the template above to slowly introduce any prebiotic supplement. I suggest buying a food scale that is capable of 1 grams measurements and I would start with 0.5 grams added to yogurt, shakes or any liquid.
- Brand: NOW Foods Organic Inulin Powder

- Note: Inulin is probably the most notorious for creating gastrointestinal distress in individuals who are not ready to supplement prebiotics; a 5 gram dose can cause a lot of discomfort.

Acacia Fiber

- See 'Inulin' information.
- Brand: NOW Foods Organic Acacia Fiber.

Potato Starch

- See 'Inulin' information.
- Brand: Bob's Red Mill Unmodified Potato Starch or Thrive Market Organic Potato Starch (not available via Fullscript).

Green Banana Flour

- See 'Inulin' information.
- Brand: NOW Foods Green Banana Flour or Let's Do Organic Green Banana Flour (not available via Fullscript).

Note: Dr. Mercola makes a product called "Organic Resistant Starch Complex", which is a perfect compilation of highly useful prebiotic fibers. I have included this in my Fullscript "GLP-1 Lifestyle" template, feel free to purchase this alone or with the other suggested prebiotic fibers in the template. This complex combines potato starch and green banana flours (alongside others), which I couldn't provide otherwise on Fullscript.

There are many commercial probiotic products available nowadays with a myriad of positive clinical results. You will be consuming probiotics in the form of yogurt, sauerkraut, etc. However, I do suggest supplementation. At first, start with single strain/species varieties which will initially turn the tide on your gut health.

Lactobacillus rhamnosus GG

• Benefits: Enhances gut health, supports immune function, balances the gut microbiome, increases level and health of commensal bacteria, improves metabolic health and GLP-1 production.
• Brand: Klaire Labs Ther-Biotic Factor 1 Probiotic

Lactobacillus gasseri BNR-17

• Benefits: 'See L. rhamnosus'. Additionally, this specifically decreases levels of visceral fat more successfully than others.
• Brand: Dr. Mercola Biothin Probiotic.

Bifidobacterium longum BB536

Benefits: 'See L. rhamnosus'.
Brand: Life Extension GI Balance.

Incorporating the right supplements can enhance GLP-1 production and support metabolic health, I have kept this list brief as supplements are only additive to an optimal lifestyle and happen to be quite expensive. These are highly studied and legitimate multipliers of your success.

Food Based "Supplements"

Ginger

• Benefits: Enhances GLP-1 production, supports digestion, supports longevity.

• Source: For all of these, I would suggest fresh, dried or powder sources and learning to utilize them in your culinary endeavors or by making tea; otherwise supplements are available and offer a medicinal dosage, which can be difficult to achieve with culinary usage.

• Dose: Can use liberally for cooking, otherwise per supplement instructions.

• Brand: Check your grocery store for fresh ginger, otherwise shredded and dried is great for tea while powder is most useful for cooking; otherwise Organic NOW Foods Ginger Root.

Cinnamon

• Benefits: Improves insulin sensitivity, supports blood sugar regulation.

• Source: See 'Ginger"

• Dose: Can use liberally for cooking, otherwise per supplement instructions.

• Brand: Cinnamon sticks are most useful for steeping and making teas and vinegars, however, powder is most useful for cooking and topping. Remember, "true" cinnamon is Ceylon cinnamon, while Cassia is considered false cinnamon. Both are actually useful for the same benefits, I suggest utilizing each. For a supplement, I have added Organic India Ceylon Cinnamon to the Fullscript template.

Fenugreek

• Benefits: Supports digestion, enhances GLP-1 production.

• Source: See 'Ginger".

• Dose: Can use liberally for cooking, otherwise per supplement instructions.

- Brand: Whole fenugreek seeds are useful for Indian dishes or making tea and stay fresher than powder forms; otherwise NOW Foods Fenugreek.
- Note: Fenugreek has the ability to increase sex hormone production and can do so potently; men, although fenugreek can and will increase testosterone production, ask your primary care provider before using a fenugreek supplement as they can cause estrogen over production and feminization.

Aloe Vera

- Benefits: Supports gut health, reduces inflammation.
- Source: Fresh juice is best, found at your grocery store.
- Dose: Consuming small amounts of aloe vera juice is the most common method, follow instructions on the bottle.
- Brand: Lily of the Desert Aloe Vera Juice.

Green Tea

- Benefits: Supports metabolic health, enhances GLP-1 production, supports longevity.
- Source: See 'Ginger".
- Dose: Can drink liberally as tea, otherwise follow supplement instructions, likely only utilizing on the Day 2 amplified fast.
- Brand: Tea must be organic as it is a highly sprayed crop, any form of green tea has many health benefits, experiment with your favorite. For a supplement, use Klaire Labs Green Tea Extract.

Core Supplements

Berberine

- Benefits: Supports blood sugar regulation and metabolic health.
- Dose: 1 gram upon waking.
- Timing: Day 2 for the amplified fast.

- Brand: Thorne Research Berberine.

Omega-3 Fatty Acids

- Benefits: Reduces inflammation, supports metabolic health.
- Dose: 3 grams upon waking and at night.
- Timing: Day 2 for the amplified fast and prior to bedtime.
- Brand: Carlson Labs Super Omega Gems.

Curcumin

- Benefits: Anti-inflammatory, supports metabolic health.
- Dose: 1-2 grams upon waking and every 4 hours if experiencing soreness or inflammation.
- Timing: Day 2 for the amplified fast.
- Brand: Thorne Curcumin Phytosome.
- Note: This entire Day 2 Amplified Fast stack can be taken the day after a rigorous exercise session when you are feeling very sore; this helps to restore muscle health and youthfulness.

Magnesium

- Benefits: Supports insulin sensitivity and metabolic health.
- Dose: 300 mg, four days per week.
- Timing: Ideally taken in the evening to support relaxation and sleep.
- Brand: Klaire Labs Magnesium Glycinate Complex.

Alpha-Lipoic Acid (ALA)

- Benefits: Supports insulin sensitivity and metabolic health.
- Dose: 600 mg per day up to 3 days per week.
- Timing: Take just prior to meals.
- Brand: Thorne Alpha-Lipoic Acid.

Optional Supplements, if desired and budget allows:

Bitter Melon

- Benefits: Enhances glucose metabolism, supports insulin sensitivity.
- Brand: Himalaya Organic Bitter Melon.

Quercetin

- Benefits: Anti-inflammatory, supports immune function.
- Brand: NOW Foods Quercetin with Bromelain.

Ginseng

- Benefits: Supports energy levels, enhances GLP-1 production.
- Brand: NOW Foods Panax Ginseng.

Lifestyle modifications are non-negotiable and non-temporary, you need to learn to incorporate these practices into your forever routine. They are critically deficient in modern humans and in many ways, the core of our modern disease states:

Sun Exposure

- Morning Sun: Very important to circadian rhythm, digestion and hormone balance; any amount of morning sun in the eyes is better than nothing, otherwise get as much as your time allows, no need for sun protection here as UV rays are minimal until approximately 9-11 AM.
- Afternoon Sun: Learn how to build your solar tolerance by spending 20 minutes at a time in midday heat and then retreating indoors, to shade or by wearing full cover sun clothing for another period of time and continuing this cycle without allowing yourself

to burn. This builds vitamin D in an optimal way. Cold water exposure will limit sunburn potential by cooling off your skin.

- Tip: Use sun clothing instead of sunscreen to protect your skin.
- Red Light Therapy: Good way to mimic morning sun, many light panel options are available in various price ranges.

Grounding

- Practice: Spend at least 20-30 minutes daily walking barefoot on natural surfaces like grass, sand, or soil or immerse yourself in a natural body of water.

Nature Bathing

- Practice: Spend at least two hours per week immersed in nature, such as hiking in a forest, walking by a lake, or sitting in a park. Ideally, you would do it much more often than this. Watching the clouds pass in your backyard is surprisingly therapeutic.

Quality of Water

- Practice: Learn about your local water source and chlorination, fluoridation, wastewater recycling, etc; Use a Berkey filter with fluoride attachments, reverse osmosis (RO) system or drink spring water.
- Intake: Drink at least half your body weight in ounces per day. Use a product like LMNT if you want to add flavor, electrolytes and fun to your water every now and again.

Cold Exposure

- Practice: Turn your shower to cold for the last minute, gradually increasing the duration you can tolerate. Immerse yourself in natural bodies of water and stay longer than your brain wants you to. Buy a cold plunge and go all in!

• Intake: Aim for 2-3 minutes of cold exposure, 3-4 times per week.

Sleep Management

• Practice: Prioritize getting 8 hours of quality sleep each night. Quality means your brain hasn't been exposed to food, alcohol, cannabis, screens or any other artificial light for at least 2 hours.

• Tips: Establish a relaxing bedtime routine, such as drinking 'sleepy' tea varieties, avoiding heavy food and screens for two hours before sleep, creating a comfortable environment with cool temperatures, no noise and significant darkness. Try meditating in the bath or hot tub prior to bedtime.

Stress Management

- Practice: Engage in mindfulness practices, the most practical being, in my opinion, breathing exercises and meditation.
- Tip: You don't have to be a Buddhist to meditate or a professional to relax with your breath.
- Meditation: Sit in a comfortable position, close your eyes and simply imagine a bright light of happiness floating around you. Now, imagine yourself floating as the ball of light, first you move throughout your neighborhood, then your community, then your city, state, Earth and finally the universe, spreading this bright light around to everything you can see. This easy and effective meditation can take one minute or an entire day, depending how long you want to float around and enjoy.
- Breathwork: The goal of breathwork is to increase vagal nerve tone and the simplest way to do this is by increasing your exhalation compared to your inhalation. All we will do for this introduction is what is known as the 4-7-8 breath. Sit in a comfortable position similar to meditation; breathe in for 4

seconds, hold it for 7 seconds and breath out for 8 seconds. Repeat this for as long as you'd like, ideally at least 5 minutes.

Regular exercise is essential for optimizing your lifestyle. I am not going to go into any specific details here, just understand this simple fact. You need to get active, one way or another. Make it fun, make it sustainable. Aim for bits and pieces of difficult aerobic exercise (rowing), strength training (weight lifting) and easy aerobic exercise (walking). Walking should dominate while the others fill complimentary roles. Generally speaking, 150 minutes per week is a good goal.

To maintain optimal health, avoid the following additives commonly found in processed foods:

- Artificial sweeteners (aspartame, sucralose, saccharin)
- High-fructose corn syrup
- Trans fats and hydrogenated oils
- Monosodium glutamate (MSG)
- Artificial colors and flavors
- Sodium nitrites and nitrates
- Potassium bromate
- Propyl gallate
- Butylated hydroxyanisole (BHA) and butylated hydroxytoluene (BHT)
- Azodicarbonamide
- Carrageenan
- Sulfites
- Polysorbates
- Brominated vegetable oil (BVO)

- Tert-Butylhydroquinone (TBHQ)
- Acesulfame Potassium (Ace-K)
- Sodium Benzoate
- Propylene Glycol
- Parabens (methylparaben, propylparaben)
- Calcium Propionate
- Dimethylpolysiloxane

This chapter details the most important facts covered in this entire book. Save it, re-read it, most importantly, get to practice! Understand the importance of recognizing side effects of semaglutide, using a structured eating pattern for GLP-1 optimization, and the inclusion of key foods and fiber in your diet. The benefits of specific probiotics and supplements for enhancing GLP-1 production cannot be overstated. Additionally, the significance of lifestyle practices such as sun exposure, grounding, nature bathing, quality water intake, cold exposure, regular exercise, and effective sleep and stress management will improve your life in more ways than you could yet fully realize.

CONCLUSION

Thank you for joining me on this transformative journey through "The GLP-1 Lifestyle." Your dedication to understanding and optimizing your metabolic health is truly commendable, and I am grateful for your trust and commitment.

As you reflect on the information and strategies presented in this book, remember that achieving and maintaining a healthy weight is a lifelong journey. It is not about perfection, but about progress and persistence. There will be challenges and setbacks along the way, but with the right tools and mindset, you can overcome them and achieve your health goals.

Stay committed to the daily eating patterns, the incorporation of key foods, and the structured lifestyle practices outlined in this book. These strategies are not just about weight loss, but about fostering a sustainable and healthy lifestyle that promotes overall well-being. Remember, your health journey is unique, and it's important to find what works best for you and to adapt the strategies to fit your individual needs.

I encourage you to seek support and build a community around your health journey. Join my Facebook group, "The GLP-1 Lifestyle," where you can connect with others who are on the same path, share your experiences, and find encouragement and motivation, as well as speak to me directly with any problems you are facing.

The future of your health is bright, and I am incredibly optimistic about the transformation you will achieve. Embrace the GLP-1 lifestyle with confidence and enthusiasm, knowing that you have the power to create lasting change. Look forward to a healthier, happier, and more vibrant life, filled with energy and vitality. Thank you for allowing me to be a part of your journey. Your success and well-being are at the heart of this book, and I am honored to have shared this knowledge with you. Here's to your continued progress and the incredible health transformations that await you. Stay committed, stay inspired, and embrace the journey with open arms. Your best self is within reach, and I believe in your ability to achieve greatness. Cheers to your health and happiness!

For the Journey,

Dr. Hackett

REFERENCES

SECTION I

1. Bray, G. A., & Ryan, D. H. (2021). Update on obesity pharmacotherapy. *Annals of the New York Academy of Sciences*, 1464(1), 72-85.
2. Rosenbaum, M., & Leibel, R. L. (2010). Adaptive thermogenesis in humans. *International Journal of Obesity*, 34(S1), S47-S55.
3. Ludwig, D. S., & Ebbeling, C. B. (2018). The carbohydrate-insulin model of obesity: beyond "calories in, calories out". *JAMA Internal Medicine*, 178(8), 1098-1103.
4. Hall, K. D., Kahan, S., & Catenacci, V. A. (2020). Strategies for sustainable weight loss: from diet to dietary patterns. *Mayo Clinic Proceedings*, 95(2), 316-324.
5. MacLean, P. S., Higgins, J. A., Giles, E. D., Sherk, V. D., & Jackman, M. R. (2015). The role for adipose tissue in weight regain after weight loss. *Obesity Reviews*, 16(S1), 45-54.
6. Sumithran, P., Prendergast, L. A., Delbridge, E., Purcell, K., Shulkes, A., Kriketos, A., & Proietto, J. (2011). Long-term persistence of hormonal adaptations to weight loss. *New England Journal of Medicine*, 365(17), 1597-1604.
7. Gerstein, H. C., Colhoun, H. M., Dagenais, G. R., Díaz, R., Lakshmanan, M., Pais, P., ... & Basile, J. (2019). Dulaglutide and cardiovascular outcomes in type 2 diabetes (REWIND): a double-blind, randomised placebo-controlled trial. *The Lancet*, 394(10193), 121-130.
8. Wilding, J. P. H., et al. (2021). Once-Weekly Semaglutide in Adults with Overweight or Obesity. *The New England Journal of Medicine*, 384(11), 989-1002.
9. Davies, M., et al. (2022). Semaglutide 2.4 mg once a week in adults with overweight or obesity: the STEP 1 trial. *The Lancet*, 399(10338), 1821-1832.
10. Zheng, Y., Ley, S. H., & Hu, F. B. (2018). Global aetiology and epidemiology of type 2 diabetes mellitus and its complications. Nature Reviews Endocrinology, 14(2), 88-98.
11. Yanovski, S. Z., & Yanovski, J. A. (2014). Long-term drug treatment for obesity: a systematic and clinical review. JAMA, 311(1), 74-86.
12. Baggio, L. L., & Drucker, D. J. (2007). Biology of Incretins: GLP-1 and GIP. *Gastroenterology*, 132(6), 2131-2157.
13. Holst, J. J. (2007). The physiology of glucagon-like peptide 1. *Physiological Reviews*, 87(4), 1409-1439.
14. Campbell, J. E., & Drucker, D. J. (2013). Pharmacology, physiology, and mechanisms of action of incretin hormones. *Cell Metabolism*, 17(6), 819-837.

Non-Academic Sources

1. Elon Musk: Tweet about fasting and Wegovy: Twitter; Interview with the Full Send Podcast: YouTube (August 2023)
2. Oprah Winfrey: Interview with People magazine: People (January 2023)
3. Tracy Morgan: Interview on the "Today" show: YouTube (March 2023)
4. Jodi's Semaglutide Success: Triumph Over Temptation: ABC News
5. "Novo Nordisk Finds Patients Using Wegovy Keep Weight Off For 4 Years," (SurvivorNet) .
6. "Elon Musk Rockets Weight-Loss Drug Into Public Eye," (CU Anschutz Newsroom) .
7. "Elon Musk says he used a popular weight-loss drug to get 'fit, ripped, and healthy'," (Yahoo) .

8. "How do Billionaires Lose Weight Fast? Elon Musk Says Semaglutide Helped him Slim Down,"(the biostation) .
9. "Novo Nordisk's Wegovy gets a surprise endorsement from Elon Musk," (Fierce Pharma) .

SECTION II

1. Astrup, A., Carraro, R., Finer, N., Harper, A., Kolotkin, R. L., Lean, M. E., … & Wilding, J. P. (2022). Effect of once-weekly semaglutide on appetite, energy intake, control of eating, food preference and body weight in subjects with obesity. *Diabetes, Obesity and Metabolism*, 24(8), 1653-1666.
2. Ueda, Y., Yamada, Y., & Seino, Y. (2020). The role of gut hormones in glucose homeostasis. *Journal of Diabetes Investigation*, 11(2), 226-237.
3. Drucker, D. J. (2018). The cardiovascular biology of glucagon-like peptide-1. Cell Metabolism, 27(3), 531-545.
4. Lau, J., Bloch, P., Schaffer, L., Konkle, B., Lam, N., Lee, A., ... & Maahs, D. M. (2022). Effect of semaglutide treatment on body weight and energy expenditure in people with overweight or obesity: a randomized clinical trial. JAMA, 328(15), 1497-1507.
5. Davies, M. J., Bergenstal, R. M., Bode, B., DeFronzo, R. A., Eldor, R., Inzucchi, S. E., ... & Rosenstock, J. (2018). Efficacy of Liraglutide for weight loss among patients with type 2 diabetes: the SCALE Obesity and Prediabetes NN8022-1839 Trial. JAMA, 324(7), 635-645.
6. Le Roux, C. W., & Bloom, S. R. (2005). Gut-brain interactions in appetite regulation. Comprehensive Physiology, 5(1), 13-30.
7. Nauck, M. A., Meier, J. J., Cavender, M. A., Abd El Aziz, M., Raben, A., Pontiroli, A. E., ... & Holst, J. J. (2016). Gastric inhibitory polypeptide and glucagon-like peptide-1 in the pathogenesis of type 2 diabetes. Diabetes, 65(12), 3651-3669.
8. Feinsinger, A., et al. (2016). Seasonal variation in gut hormone levels in healthy adults. The Journal of Clinical Endocrinology & Metabolism, 101(5), 2063-2070.
9. Saeed, M. I., et al. (2021). The impact of sunlight exposure on gut microbiota and metabolic health: A systematic review. Critical Reviews in Food Science and Nutrition, 61(18), 3014-3026.
10. Kahn, S. E., et al. (2001). The incretin effect and insulin resistance: implications for the treatment of type 2 diabetes mellitus. Endocrine Reviews, 22(5), 588-613.
11. Nogueiras, R., et al. (2012). The gut microbiota regulates diurnal rhythms of GLP-1 secretion in mice. Molecular Metabolism, 1(4), 364-373.
12. Stenlöf, K., et al. (2019). Gut hormones and exercise: effects on energy balance and metabolism. Journal of Endocrinology, 242(1), R65-R83.
13. Levin, G. A., et al. (2023). Effect of sunlight exposure on GLP-1 secretion and glucose metabolism in healthy adults. Diabetes Care, 46(1), 123-130.
14. Chambers, A. P., & Sandoval, D. A. (2021). The role of the gut microbiome in obesity and metabolic disease. Current Obesity Reports, 10(4), 316-324.
15. Burcelin, R., et al. (2017). Gut microbiota and immune crosstalk in metabolic disease. Molecular Metabolism, 6(9), 1107-1119.
16. Zheng, D., Liwinski, T., & Elinav, E. (2020). Interaction between microbiota and immunity in health and disease. Cell Research, 30(6), 492-506.

Non-Academic Sources:

1. National Institutes of Health (NIH). (2023). Gastrointestinal Side Effects of GLP-1 Agonists. Available from: NIH Gastrointestinal Side Effects
2. Medscape. (2023). Managing GI Side Effects of GLP-1 Agonists. Available from: Medscape GI Side Effects

3. FDA. (2023). Drug Safety Communication: Risk of Pancreatitis with GLP-1 Agonists. Available from: FDA Pancreatitis Risk
4. New England Journal of Medicine (NEJM). (2023). Gallbladder-Related Side Effects of GLP-1 Agonists. Available from: NEJM Gallbladder Side Effects
5. SUSTAIN-6 Trial. (2016). Semaglutide and Diabetic Retinopathy Outcomes. Available from: SUSTAIN-6 Trial
6. National Cancer Institute (NCI). (2023). Medullary Thyroid Carcinoma and GLP-1 Agonists. Available from: NCI Medullary Thyroid Carcinoma
7. PubMed. (2023). Systematic Review and Meta-Analysis of GLP-1 Agonist Side Effects. Available from: PubMed Systematic Review
8. ClinicalTrials.gov. (2023). Adverse Events in GLP-1 Agonist Studies. Available from: ClinicalTrials.gov Adverse Events

SECTION III

1. SUSTAIN 6: A long-term clinical trial comparing Ozempic to other diabetes medications, demonstrating significant reductions in HbA1c and the risk of kidney disease progression.
2. Apovian, C. M. (2022). The GLP-1 receptor agonists: A new era in the treatment of obesity. The American Journal of Managed Care, 28(12 Spec No.), S457-S465.
3. Lingvay, I., Pi-Sunyer, X., Wilding, J. P., Langkilde, A. M., Baquero, A. F., Bergenstal, R. M., ... & Rosenstock, J. (2022). Efficacy and safety of semaglutide 2.4 mg for weight management in adults with overweight or obesity: the STEP 5 trial. JAMA, 327(7), 609-620.
4. Wadden, T. A., Womble, L. G., Tsai, A. G., Smith, S. R., Aronne, L. J., & McLaughlin, T. (2020). Weight maintenance and additional weight loss with liraglutide after low-calorie-diet-induced weight loss: the SCALE Maintenance randomized clinical trial. International Journal of Obesity, 44(10), 2054-2066.
5. Marso, S. P., Bain, S. C., Consoli, A., et al. (2016). Semaglutide and Cardiovascular Outcomes in Patients with Type 2 Diabetes. New England Journal of Medicine, 375, 1834-1844.
6. Pratley, R. E., Aroda, V. R., Lingvay, I., et al. (2018). Semaglutide Versus Dulaglutide Once Weekly in Patients with Type 2 Diabetes (SUSTAIN 7): A Randomised, Open-Label, Phase 3b Trial. Lancet Diabetes Endocrinology, 6(4), 275-286.
7. Rosenstock, J., Allison, D., Birkenfeld, A. L., et al. (2019). Effect of Additional Oral Semaglutide vs Sitagliptin on Glycated Hemoglobin in Adults with Type 2 Diabetes: The PIONEER 3 Randomized Clinical Trial. JAMA, 321(15), 1466-1480.
8. Goldenberg, R. M., & Steen, O. (2019). Semaglutide: Review and Place in Therapy for Adults with Type 2 Diabetes. Canadian Journal of Diabetes, 43(2), 136-145.
9. Holst, J. J., & Deacon, C. F. (2013). Is There a Place for Inhibitors of Dipeptidyl Peptidase IV in the Treatment of Type 2 Diabetes Mellitus? Drugs, 57(1), 7-10.
10. Nyberg, J., Jacobsen, L. V., & Bethel, A. (2016). Cardiovascular Safety of Semaglutide in Subjects with Type 2 Diabetes: A Meta-Analysis. Cardiovascular Diabetology, 15, 23.
11. Pereira, M. J., Eriksson, J. W. (2019). Emerging Role of SGLT-2 Inhibitors for the Treatment of Obesity. Drugs, 79(3), 219-230.
12. Sattar, N., McGuire, D. K., et al. (2021). Effects of Glucagon-like Peptide-1 Receptor Agonists on Cardiovascular Outcomes in Patients with Type 2 Diabetes: A Meta-Analysis of Randomised Controlled Trials. Lancet Diabetes Endocrinology, 9(10), 653-662.

13. Wadden, T. A., Bailey, T. S., Billings, L. K., et al. (2021). Effect of Subcutaneous Semaglutide vs Placebo as an Adjunct to Intensive Behavioral Therapy on Body Weight in Adults with Overweight or Obesity: The STEP 3 Randomized Clinical Trial. JAMA, 325(14), 1403-1413.
14. Guthrie, R. A., & Guthrie, D. W. (2004). Pathophysiology of Diabetes Mellitus. Critical Care Nursing Quarterly, 27(2), 113-125.
15. Kapitza, C., Forst, T., Coester, H. V., et al. (2013). Pharmacodynamics and Pharmacokinetics of Semaglutide in Healthy Subjects and Subjects with Type 2 Diabetes. Diabetes, Obesity and Metabolism, 15(5), 406-414.
16. Matthews, D. R., Paldánius, P. M., Proot, P., et al. (2018). Glycaemic Efficacy and Safety of Once-weekly Semaglutide Versus Exenatide Extended Release in Subjects with Type 2 Diabetes (SUSTAIN 3): A Multicentre, Double-blind, Randomised, Parallel-group, Phase 3a Trial. Lancet Diabetes Endocrinology, 6(4), 275-286.
17. Weinstock, R. S., & Lavery, B. (2020). Management of Type 2 Diabetes in Older Adults: Special Considerations. Diabetes Spectrum, 33(3), 218-225.
18. Blonde, L., & Stenlöf, K. (2020). Glucagon-like Peptide-1 Receptor Agonists for Type 2 Diabetes. Diabetes Spectrum, 33(4), 351-360.
19. Rubino, D. M., Greenway, F. L., Khalid, U., et al. (2021). Effect of Weekly Subcutaneous Semaglutide vs Daily Liraglutide on Weight Loss in Adults with Overweight or Obesity: The STEP 8 Randomized Clinical Trial. JAMA, 325(14), 1410-1420.
20. Rosenstock, J., Wysham, C., Frías, J. P., et al. (2019). Efficacy and Safety of Injectable Semaglutide Once Weekly Versus Sitagliptin Once Daily in Patients with Type 2 Diabetes (SUSTAIN 2): A Phase 3a, Randomised, Double-blind, Double-dummy, Placebo- and Active-controlled Trial. Lancet Diabetes Endocrinology, 5(4), 341-354.

Non-Academic Sources

1. American Diabetes Association. (2020). Standards of Medical Care in Diabetes—2020. Diabetes Care, 43(Suppl 1), S1-S212.
2. American Diabetes Association. (2020). Pharmacologic Approaches to Glycemic Treatment: Standards of Medical Care in Diabetes—2020. Diabetes Care, 43(Suppl 1), S98-S110.
3. ADA Standards of Care 2021. (2021). Standards of Medical Care in Diabetes—2021. Diabetes Care, 44(Suppl 1), S1-S232.

SECTION IV

1. Hartmann, K., et al. (2021). Anti-diabetic treatment leads to changes in gut microbiome. Frontiers in Bioengineering and Biotechnology, 24.
2. Zhang, Z., et al. (2023). Semaglutide alleviates gut microbiota dysbiosis induced by a high-fat diet. BMC Microbiology, 23(1), 1-13.
3. Zhao, Y., et al. (2023). Effects of semaglutide on the gut microbiota and intestinal barrier in patients with obesity and type 2 diabetes mellitus. Journal of Diabetes Research, 2023.
4. Tilg, H., & Moschen, A. R. (2017). Microbiota and metabolism: role in obesity and metabolic disease. Gut, 66(8), 1436-1444.
5. Cao, J., et al. (2022). Effects of Glucagon-like Peptide-1 Receptor Agonists on Gut Microbiota in Obesity and Type 2 Diabetes: A Systematic Review. Frontiers in Endocrinology, 13.
6. Liu, Y., et al. (2023). Semaglutide Improves Gut Microbiota Dysbiosis in Obese Mice by Activating the GLP-1R/AMPK Signaling Pathway. Journal of Diabetes Research, 2023.
7. Duan, X., et al. (2024). Semaglutide alleviates gut microbiota dysbiosis induced by a high-fat diet. European Journal of Pharmacology, 969, 176440.

8. Gibson, G.R., et al. (2017). Dietary prebiotics: current status and new definition. Food Science and Technology Bulletin: Functional Foods, 7(1), 1-19. DOI: 10.1616/1476-2137.15880.
9. Slavin, J. (2013). Fiber and prebiotics: mechanisms and health benefits. Nutrients, 5(4), 1417-1435. DOI: 10.3390/nu5041417.
10. Roberfroid, M., et al. (2010). Prebiotic effects: metabolic and health benefits. British Journal of Nutrition, 104(S2), S1-S63. DOI: 10.1017/S0007114510003363.
11. Scott, K.P., et al. (2013). The influence of diet on the gut microbiota. Pharmacological Research, 69(1), 52-60. DOI: 10.1016/j.phrs.2012.10.020.
12. Davani-Davari, D., Negahdaripour, M., Karimzadeh, I., Seifan, M., Mohkam, M., Masoumi, S.J., Berenjian, A., & Ghasemi, Y. (2019). Prebiotics: Definition, Types, Sources, Mechanisms, and Clinical Applications. Foods, 8(3), 92. DOI: 10.3390/foods8030092.
13. Kolida, S., & Gibson, G.R. (2007). Prebiotic capacity of inulin-type fructans. Journal of Nutrition, 137(11 Suppl), 2503S-2506S. DOI: 10.1093/jn/137.11.2503S.
14. Swanson, K.S., et al. (2020). The International Scientific Association for Probiotics and Prebiotics (ISAPP) consensus statement on the definition and scope of prebiotics. Nature Reviews Gastroenterology & Hepatology, 17, 687–701. DOI: 10.1038/s41575-020-0344-2.
15. Tandon, D., Haque, M.M., & Mande, S.S. (2010). Identification of Bacterial Species Associated with Wheat and Rice Crop Rhizospheres from Sites in India. Current Science, 99(10), 1384-1388. URL: http://www.jstor.org/stable/24077007.
16. Hill, C., et al. (2014). Expert consensus document: The International Scientific Association for Probiotics and Prebiotics consensus statement on the scope and appropriate use of the term probiotic. Nature Reviews Gastroenterology & Hepatology, 11, 506–514. DOI: 10.1038/nrgastro.2014.66.
17. Ouwehand, A.C., et al. (2010). Probiotics: mechanisms and established effects. International Dairy Journal, 20(10), 753-761. DOI: 10.1016/j.idairyj.2010.06.001.
18. Sanders, M.E., et al. (2018). Probiotics for human use. Nutrition Bulletin, 43(3), 212-225. DOI: 10.1111/nbu.12334.
19. Plaza-Diaz, J., Ruiz-Ojeda, F.J., Vilchez-Padial, L.M., & Gil, A. (2019). Evidence of the Anti-Inflammatory Effects of Probiotics and Synbiotics in Intestinal Chronic Diseases. Nutrients, 11(2), 293. DOI: 10.3390/nu11020293.
20. Gopal, P.K., & Gill, H.S. (2000). Oligosaccharides and glycoconjugates in bovine milk and colostrum. British Journal of Nutrition, 84(S1), 69-74. DOI: 10.1017/S0007114500002159.
21. Hemarajata, P., & Versalovic, J. (2013). Effects of probiotics on gut microbiota: mechanisms of intestinal immunomodulation and neuromodulation. Therapeutic Advances in Gastroenterology, 6(1), 39-51. DOI: 10.1177/1756283X12459294.
22. Sanders, M.E. (2009). How do we know when something called "probiotic" is really a probiotic? A guideline for consumers and health care professionals. Functional Food Reviews, 1(3), 3-12. URL: https://pubmed.ncbi.nlm.nih.gov/24669186/.
23. Sonnenburg, J.L., & Bäckhed, F. (2016). Diet–microbiota interactions as moderators of human metabolism. Nature, 535, 56
24. Plaza-Diaz, J., Ruiz-Ojeda, F.J., Vilchez-Padial, L.M., & Gil, A. (2019). Evidence of the Anti-Inflammatory Effects of Probiotics and Synbiotics in Intestinal Chronic Diseases. Nutrients, 11(2), 293. DOI: 10.3390/nu11020293.
25. Wegh, C.A.M., Geerlings, S.Y., Knol, J., Roeselers, G., & Belzer, C. (2019). Postbiotics and Their Potential Applications in Early Life Nutrition and Beyond. International Journal of Molecular Sciences, 20(19), 4673. DOI: 10.3390/ijms20194673.

26. Ríos-Covián, D., Ruas-Madiedo, P., Margolles, A., Gueimonde, M., de los Reyes-Gavilán, C.G., & Salazar, N. (2016). Intestinal Short Chain Fatty Acids and their Link with Diet and Human Health. Frontiers in Microbiology, 7, 185. DOI: 10.3389/fmicb.2016.00185.
27. Arpaia, N., Campbell, C., Fan, X., Dikiy, S., van der Veeken, J., deRoos, P., Liu, H., Cross, J.R., Pfeffer, K., Coffer, P.J., Rudensky, A.Y. (2013). Metabolites produced by commensal bacteria promote peripheral regulatory T-cell generation. Nature, 504, 451-455. DOI: 10.1038/nature12726.
28. Tan, J., McKenzie, C., Potamitis, M., Thorburn, A.N., Mackay, C.R., & Macia, L. (2014). The role of short-chain fatty acids in health and disease. Advances in Immunology, 121, 91-119. DOI: 10.1016/B978-0-12-800100-4.00003-9.
29. Koh, A., De Vadder, F., Kovatcheva-Datchary, P., & Bäckhed, F. (2016). From Dietary Fiber to Host Physiology: Short-Chain Fatty Acids as Key Bacterial Metabolites. Cell, 165(6), 1332-1345. DOI: 10.1016/j.cell.2016.05.041.
30. Markowiak-Kopeć, P., & Śliżewska, K. (2020). The effect of probiotics on the production of short-chain fatty acids by human intestinal microbiome. Nutrients, 12(4), 1107. DOI: 10.3390/nu12041107.
31. Canfora, E.E., Meex, R.C.R., Venema, K., & Blaak, E.E. (2019). Gut microbial metabolites in obesity, NAFLD, and T2DM. Nature Reviews Endocrinology, 15, 261-273. DOI: 10.1038/s41574-019-0156-z.
32. Lucas, R. M., & Ponsonby, A. L. (2002). Ultraviolet radiation and health: friend and foe. Medical Journal of Australia, 177(11-12), 594-598. DOI: 10.5694/j.1326-5377.2002.tb04930.x
33. Holick, M. F. (2007). Vitamin D deficiency. New England Journal of Medicine, 357(3), 266-281.DOI: 10.1056/NEJMra070553
34. Cantorna, M. T., Snyder, L., Lin, Y. D., & Yang, L. (2015). Vitamin D and 1,25(OH)2D regulation of T cells. Nutrients, 7(4), 3011-3021. DOI: 10.3390/nu7043011
35. Oschman, J. L. (2007). Can electrons act as antioxidants? A review and commentary. Journal of Alternative and Complementary Medicine, 13(9), 955-967.DOI: 10.1089/acm.2007.7048
36. Chevalier, G., Sinatra, S. T., Oschman, J. L., Delany, R. M., & Karabanow, H. S. (2012). Earthing (grounding) the human body reduces blood viscosity—a major factor in cardiovascular disease. Journal of Alternative and Complementary Medicine, 19(2), 102-110.DOI: 10.1089/acm.2011.0820
37. Jadhav, S. V., Bringas, E., Yadav, G. D., Rathod, V. K., Ortiz, I., & Marathe, K. V. (2015). Arsenic and fluoride contaminated groundwaters: a review of current technologies for contaminants removal. Journal of Environmental Management, 162, 306-325.DOI: 10.1016/j.jenvman.2015.07.020
38. Singh, A., Kumar, A., & Sharma, A. (2018). Fluoride ions vs removal technologies: A study. Journal of Environmental Chemical Engineering, 6(3), 3521-3533.DOI: 10.1016/j.jece.2018.05.042
39. Benbrook, C. M. (2016). Trends in glyphosate herbicide use in the United States and globally. Environmental Sciences Europe, 28(1), 3.DOI: 10.1186/s12302-016-0070-0
40. Mostafalou, S., & Abdollahi, M. (2017). Pesticides and human chronic diseases: Evidences, mechanisms, and perspectives. Toxicology and Applied Pharmacology, 297, 37-41.DOI: 10.1016/j.taap.2016.12.011
41. Stevens, L. J., Kuczek, T., Burgess, J. R., Hurt, E., & Arnold, L. E. (2010). Dietary sensitivities and ADHD symptoms: thirty-five years of research. Clinical Pediatrics, 50(4), 279-293. DOI: 10.1177/0009922810384728
42. Bateman, B., Warner, J. O., Hutchinson, E., Dean, T., Rowlandson, P., Gant, C., … & Stevenson, J. (2004). The effects of a double blind, placebo controlled, artificial food colourings and benzoate preservative challenge on hyperactivity in a general population sample of preschool children. Archives of Disease in Childhood, 89(6), 506-511.DOI: 10.1136/adc.2003.031435

43. Pedersen, B. K., & Saltin, B. (2015). Exercise as medicine–evidence for prescribing exercise as therapy in 26 different chronic diseases. Scandinavian Journal of Medicine & Science in Sports, 25(S3), 1-72.DOI: 10.1111/sms.12581
44. Warburton, D. E., Nicol, C. W., & Bredin, S. S. (2006). Health benefits of physical activity: the evidence. Canadian Medical Association Journal, 174(6), 801-809.DOI: 10.1503/cmaj.051351
45. Park, B. J., Tsunetsugu, Y., Kasetani, T., Kagawa, T., & Miyazaki, Y. (2010). The physiological effects of Shinrin-yoku (taking in the forest atmosphere or forest bathing): evidence from field experiments in 24 forests across Japan. Environmental Health and Preventive Medicine, 15(1), 18-26.DOI: 10.1007/s12199-009-0086-9
46. Li, Q. (2010). Effect of forest bathing trips on human immune function. Environmental Health and Preventive Medicine, 15(1), 9-17.DOI: 10.1007/s12199-008-0068-3

SECTION V

1. Bindels, L. B., Delzenne, N. M., Cani, P. D., & Walter, J. (2015). Towards a more comprehensive concept for prebiotics. Nature Reviews Gastroenterology & Hepatology, 12(5), 303-310.
2. Farooqi, I. S., & O'Rahilly, S. (2009). Leptin: a pivotal regulator of human energy homeostasis. The American Journal of Clinical Nutrition, 89(3), 980S-984S.
3. Westerterp-Plantenga, M. S., Lemmens, S. G., & Westerterp, K. R. (2012). Dietary protein – its role in satiety, energetics, weight loss and health. British Journal of Nutrition, 108(S2), S105-S112.
4. Calder, P. C. (2010). Omega-3 fatty acids and inflammatory processes: from molecules to man. Biochemical Society Transactions, 38(1), 211-222. https://doi.org/10.1042/BST0380211
5. Wall, R., Ross, R. P., Fitzgerald, G. F., & Stanton, C. (2010). Fatty acids from fish: the anti-inflammatory potential of long-chain omega-3 fatty acids. Nutrition Reviews, 68(5), 280-289. https://doi.org/10.1111/j.1753-4887.2010.00287.x
6. Drucker, D. J. (2018). Mechanisms of Action and Therapeutic Application of Glucagon-like Peptide-1. Cell Metabolism, 27(4), 740-756. https://doi.org/10.1016/j.cmet.2018.03.001
7. Holst, J. J., & Madsbad, S. (2016). Mechanisms of surgical control of type 2 diabetes: GLP-1 is key factor. Surgery for Obesity and Related Diseases, 12(6), 1236-1242. https://doi.org/10.1016/j.soard.2016.02.027
8. Levine, B., & Kroemer, G. (2008). Autophagy in the pathogenesis of disease. Cell, 132(1), 27-42. https://doi.org/10.1016/j.cell.2007.12.018
9. Madeo, F., & Kroemer, G. (2019). Dietary restriction-induced autophagy: a mechanistic link between longevity and healthspan. Current Opinion in Cell Biology, 61, 117-125. https://doi.org/10.1016/j.ceb.2019.11.001
10. Holst, J. J., & Madsbad, S. (2016). Mechanisms of action of GLP-1 receptor agonists and implications for clinical practice. Diabetes, Obesity and Metabolism, 18(1), 3-8. https://doi.org/10.1111/dom.12502
11. Mattson, M. P., Longo, V. D., & Harvie, M. (2017). Impact of intermittent fasting on health and disease processes. Ageing Research Reviews, 39, 46-58. https://doi.org/10.1016/j.arr.2016.10.005
12. Sutton, E. F., Beyl, R., Early, K. S., Cefalu, W. T., Ravussin, E., & Peterson, C. M. (2018). Early time-restricted feeding improves insulin sensitivity, blood pressure, and oxidative stress even without weight loss in men with prediabetes. Cell Metabolism, 27(6), 1212-1221.e3. https://doi.org/10.1016/j.cmet.2018.04.010
13. Solon-Biet, S. M., McMahon, A. C., Ballard, J. W., Ruohonen, K., Wu, L. E., Cogger, V. C., ... & Simpson, S. J. (2014). The ratio of macronutrients, not caloric intake, dictates cardiometabolic health, aging, and longevity in ad libitum-fed mice. Cell Metabolism, 19(3), 418-430. https://doi.org/10.1016/j.cmet.2014.02.009

14. Jakubowicz, D., Barnea, M., Wainstein, J., & Froy, O. (2013). High caloric intake at breakfast vs. dinner differentially influences weight loss of overweight and obese women. Obesity, 21(12), 2504-2512. https://doi.org/10.1002/oby.20460

15. Garaulet, M., Gómez-Abellán, P., Alburquerque-Béjar, J. J., Lee, Y. C., Ordovás, J. M., & Scheer, F. A. (2013). Timing of food intake predicts weight loss effectiveness. International Journal of Obesity, 37(4), 604-611. https://doi.org/10.1038/ijo.2012.229

16. Holick, M. F. (2007). Vitamin D deficiency. New England Journal of Medicine, 357(3), 266-281. https://doi.org/10.1056/NEJMra070553

17. Wacker, M., & Holick, M. F. (2013). Sunlight and Vitamin D: A global perspective for health. Dermato-endocrinology, 5(1), 51-108. https://doi.org/10.4161/derm.24494

18. Chevalier, G., Sinatra, S. T., Oschman, J. L., Delany, R. M., & Brezinski, P. G. (2012). Earthing: Health implications of reconnecting the human body to the Earth's surface electrons. Journal of Environmental and Public Health, 2012, 291541. https://doi.org/10.1155/2012/291541

19. Oschman, J. L., Chevalier, G., & Brown, R. (2015). The effects of grounding (earthing) on inflammation, the immune response, wound healing, and prevention and treatment of chronic inflammatory and autoimmune diseases. Journal of Inflammation Research, 8, 83-96. https://doi.org/10.2147/JIR.S69656

20. Van der Lans, A. A., Hoeks, J., Brans, B., Vijgen, G. H., Visser, M. G., Vosselman, M. J., … & Schrauwen, P. (2013). Cold acclimation recruits human brown fat and increases nonshivering thermogenesis. Journal of Clinical Investigation, 123(8), 3395-3403. https://doi.org/10.1172/JCI68993

21. Celi, F. S. (2010). Brown adipose tissue—when it pays to be inefficient. New England Journal of Medicine, 362(25), 2333-2334. https://doi.org/10.1056/NEJMcibr1004283

22. Laukkanen, T., Kunutsor, S. K., Zaccardi, F., & Laukkanen, J. A. (2018). Acute effects of sauna bathing on cardiovascular function. Journal of Human Hypertension, 32(2), 129-130. https://doi.org/10.1038/s41371-018-0058-y

23. Rhonda P. Patrick & David E. Fisher. (2015). Benefits of Heat Shock Proteins. Cell Metabolism. https://doi.org/10.1016/j.cmet.2015.09.004

24. McEwen, B. S. (2008). Central effects of stress hormones in health and disease: Understanding the protective and damaging effects of stress and stress mediators. European Journal of Pharmacology, 583(2-3), 174-185. https://doi.org/10.1016/j.ejphar.2007.11.071

25. Chrousos, G. P. (2009). Stress and disorders of the stress system. Nature Reviews Endocrinology, 5(7), 374-381. https://doi.org/10.1038/nrendo.2009.106

26. Spiegel, K., Tasali, E., Penev, P., & Van Cauter, E. (2004). Brief communication: Sleep curtailment in healthy young men is associated with decreased leptin levels, elevated ghrelin levels, and increased hunger and appetite. Annals of Internal Medicine, 141(11), 846-850. https://doi.org/10.7326/0003-4819-141-11-200412070-00008

27. Knutson, K. L., & Van Cauter, E. (2008). Associations between sleep loss and increased risk of obesity and diabetes. Annals of the New York Academy of Sciences, 1129(1), 287-304. https://doi.org/10.1196/annals.1417.033

28. Yin, J., Xing, H., & Ye, J. (2008). Efficacy of berberine in patients with type 2 diabetes mellitus. Metabolism, 57(5), 712-718. doi:10.1016/j.metabol.2008.01.013

29. Kalupahana, N. S., Claycombe, K. J., & Moustaid-Moussa, N. (2011). (n-3) Fatty acids alleviate adipose tissue inflammation and insulin resistance: mechanistic insights. Advances in Nutrition, 2(4), 304-316. doi:10.3945/an.111.000505

30. Na, L. X., Zhang, Y. L., Li, Y., Liu, L. Y., Li, R., & Kong, T. (2013). Curcumin improves insulin resistance in skeletal muscle of rats. Nutrition, Metabolism & Cardiovascular Diseases, 23(6), 536-542. doi:10.1016/j.numecd.2012.02.006

31. Yadav, H., Lee, J. H., Lloyd, J., Walter, P., & Rane, S. G. (2013). Beneficial metabolic effects of a probiotic via butyrate-induced GLP-1 hormone secretion. Journal of Biological Chemistry, 288(35), 25088-25097. doi:10.1074/jbc.M113.452516
32. Song, K. H., & Jung, M. H. (2015). Enhanced insulin sensitivity by alpha-lipoic acid accompanies increased insulin receptor substrate 2 expression and phosphorylation in high-fat fed obese mice. Journal of Nutritional Biochemistry, 26(6), 655-662. doi:10.1016/j.jnutbio.2015.01.004
33. Nammi, S., Kim, M. S., Gavande, N. S., Li, G. Q., & Roufogalis, B. D. (2009). Regulation of body weight and metabolic syndrome by ginsenoside Rb1: Evidence from laboratory investigations. Current Pharmaceutical Biotechnology, 10(1), 74-81. doi:10.2174/138920109787048677
34. Qin, B., Panickar, K. S., & Anderson, R. A. (2010). Cinnamon: Potential Role in the Prevention of Insulin Resistance, Metabolic Syndrome, and Type 2 Diabetes. Journal of Diabetes Science and Technology, 4(3), 685-693. doi:10.1177/193229681000400324
35. Srinivasan, K. (2006). Fenugreek (Trigonella foenum-graecum): A review of health beneficial physiological effects. Food Reviews International, 22(2), 203-224. doi:10.1080/87559120600586315
36. Misawa, E., Tanaka, M., Nomaguchi, K., Yamada, M., Toida, T., & Iwatsuki, K. (2012). Oral ingestion of Aloe vera phytosterols alters hepatic gene expression profiles and ameliorates obesity-associated metabolic disorders in Zucker diabetic fatty rats. Journal of Agricultural and Food Chemistry, 60(11), 2799-2806. doi:10.1021/jf2047184
37. Chaturvedi, P. (2012). Antidiabetic potentials of Momordica charantia: Multiple mechanisms behind the effects. Journal of Medicinal Food, 15(2), 101-107. doi:10.1089/jmf.2011.1947
38. Rivera, L., Morón, R., Sánchez, M., Zarzuelo, A., & Galisteo, M. (2008). Quercetin ameliorates metabolic syndrome and improves the inflammatory status in obese Zucker rats. Obesity, 16(9), 2081-2087. doi:10.1038/oby.2008.34
39. Kim, K., Park, J. M., Kim, E. H., & Han, Y. (2009). Ginsenosides Rh2 and Rg3 inhibit glucose uptake in L6 myotubes via the induction of insulin resistance and the suppression of the PDK1/Akt pathway. Archives of Pharmacal Research, 32(1), 23-28. doi:10.1007/s12272-009-1134-6
40. Wolfram, S., Raederstorff, D., Wang, Y., Teixeira, S. R., Elste, V., & Weber, P. (2005). TEAVIGO (epigallocatechin gallate) supplementation prevents obesity in mice. European Journal of Clinical Nutrition, 59(9), 1091-1097. doi:10.1038/sj.ejcn.1602224
41. Joel Greene "The Immunity Code"

SECTION VI

1. Drucker, D. J. (2018). Mechanisms of Action and Therapeutic Application of Glucagon-like Peptide-1. Cell Metabolism, 27(4), 740-756.
2. Holst, J. J., & Madsbad, S. (2016). Mechanisms of surgical control of type 2 diabetes: GLP-1 is key factor. Surgery for Obesity and Related Diseases, 12(6), 1236-1242.
3. Levine, B., & Kroemer, G. (2008). Autophagy in the pathogenesis of disease. Cell, 132(1), 27-42.
4. Madeo, F., & Kroemer, G. (2019). Dietary restriction-induced autophagy: a mechanistic link between longevity and healthspan. Current Opinion in Cell Biology, 61, 117-125.
5. Drucker, D. J. (2018). Mechanisms of action and therapeutic application of glucagon-like peptide-1. Cell Metabolism, 27(4), 740-756.
6. Holst, J. J., & Madsbad, S. (2016). Mechanisms of action of GLP-1 receptor agonists and implications for clinical practice. Diabetes, Obesity and Metabolism, 18(1), 3-8.
7. Mattson, M. P., Longo, V. D., & Harvie, M. (2017). Impact of intermittent fasting on health and disease processes. Ageing Research Reviews, 39, 46-58.

8.